The
Fasting
Diet

The Fasting Diet

A PRACTICAL FIVE-DAY PROGRAM FOR INCREASED ENERGY, GREATER STAMINA, AND A CLEARER MIND

STEVEN BAILEY, N.D.

Contemporary Books

Chicago   New York   San Francisco   Lisbon   Madrid   Mexico City   Milan
New Delhi   San Juan   Seoul   Singapore   Sydney   Toronto

Library of Congress Cataloging-in-Publication Data

Bailey, Steven, N.D.
     The fasting diet / Steven Bailey.
         p.   cm.
     Includes bibliographical references and index.
     ISBN 0-658-01145-6
     1. Fasting—Popular works.   I. Title.

    RM226.B35   2001
    613.7—dc21   2001032553

Contemporary Books

A Division of The McGraw·Hill Companies

2 3 4 5 6 7 8 9 0 AGM/AGM 0 9 8 7 6 5 4 3 2

ISBN 0-658-01145-6

This book was set in Sabon
Printed and bound by Quebecor Martinsburg

Cover design by Laurie Young
Interior design by Monica Baziuk
Interior art by Sandra Bolton

Contents

The Purpose of This Book • Why Fast? • Concepts of Health
• Stress and Disease • Spiritual Health

Normal Anatomy and Physiology of Digestion • Normal
Elimination and Removal of Toxins • Microflora Out of Balance:
Intestinal Dysbiosis • Intestinal Dysbiosis: Diagnosis
and Treatment

Preface

We live in a remarkable age. Outside of cataclysmic events of nature, we have never faced such an ever-changing environment as we do today. We have altered the natural face of the planet. We have polluted our air, land, water, and oceans like never before. Our pollutants include not only the natural wastes of the past but also a whole array of new chemicals and toxins that never existed prior to the twentieth century. Our lifestyles, diet, and especially our food sources have radically changed.

Most of these changes have been made intentionally, and with the promise of an improved quality of life behind their insertion into our world. Unfortunately, many of the results have cost us dearly. Cancer, cardiovascular disease, and a whole array of chronic disease states have followed in these footsteps. Today, more than four times as many Americans die from cancer as in 1972 when the U.S. "war on cancer" was declared.[1]

There has never been a more important time for the science of fasting to return to our personal health programs. From the standpoint of detoxification and disease reversal, fasting has no equal. I only hope that I may find the words to share my knowledge, experience, passion, and confidence in a manner that allows you to embrace this important tradition and natural practice and include it in your own life.

Acknowledgments

My life path has been truly blessed by the love and wisdom of many remarkable people. I am thankful to so many for their shared love, knowledge, and encouragement throughout my life. In this first complete work on fasting I would like to especially acknowledge and thank:

My wife, Susan, and daughter, Shayla, for their never-ending support and sacrifice during the long hours of writing.

My mother, Helen, and father, George, for the lessons and support they have provided over the years.

My primary editor and friend, Mari Florence, for making this book a reality.

My many teachers, including my students, patients, and especially:

My friends and colleagues through the years: John Bastyr, N.D.; Joseph Boucher, N.D.; Ravinder Sahni, N.D., D.C.; Bill Mitchell, N.D.; Elaine Bayes Gillaspie, N.D.; Robert Mendelson, M.D.; Diane Adler; and Bill Dyer.

And finally, those special teachers of a loving heart:

Tayeb Hayawara, a Muslim friend who worked with Gandhi and radiated love in every breath.

Leroy Vinegar, master of the jazz bass, who opened his heart and stage to so many others and me.

Douglas Kramer, nearly a doctor, who died in his last year of study with cystic fibrosis and a legacy of love, courage, and like Leroy and Tayeb, an infectious smile that lifted your spirit.

Introduction

Few areas of traditional medicine have received as much undeserved criticism as has fasting. The benefits of fasting are observable and predictable, and they serve as a remarkable example of the healing power of the human body. Regardless, contemporary authors and the press consistently ignore the positive aspects of fasting and erroneously warn about the dangers of starvation and deprivation. Fasting is neither a state of deprivation nor starvation; it is a condition of enhanced repair, rejuvenation, and healing. Hopefully this book will provide you with the knowledge to laugh at the false criticisms and to incorporate healthful fasting in your present and future practices.

It has been more than thirty years since I did my first intentional fast. Though poorly done, I nonetheless was immediately impressed by the profound physical changes that occurred when I stopped eating for more than twenty-four hours. My appetite actually decreased, my energy was good, my sense of smell and taste were remarkably enhanced, and I generally felt better than I would have expected. Over the next few years I did numerous one- and two-day fasts, typically having similar experiences, but still unaware of even the most basic guidelines for fasting.

In early 1971 I did my first supervised fast, a seven-day juice fast using primarily bottled fruit juices. I felt great throughout the juice phase and was able to keep up my normal activities including regular exercise. While I was given good information on how much juice and water to drink, I was not instructed on how to reintroduce foods, and like earlier experiences, broke the fast too abruptly. This experience, both good and bad, sent me into a lifelong journey of inquiry and practice of the art of fasting.

For the past eighteen years, I have been leading groups and individual patients on extended fasts. I never cease to be amazed by the remarkable improvements that many of my patients and group participants experience while fasting—improvements that truly speak of an enlivened body and spirit, as they represent a more focused balance, repair, and detoxification process coming from within. These improvements often represent personal freedom, a springboard toward more empowerment in the care of day-to-day and long-term health needs. When people realize that long-tolerated or medicated conditions can be positively impacted by diet, fasting, and the power of their own natural healing, their choices in life have opened immensely.

This book incorporates my own experience and that of my many patients who have fasted in my programs. It will also attempt to provide you with the knowledge necessary to safely and enthusiastically embark on your own fasting journeys. Enjoy!

The
Fasting
Diet

1

The Forgotten Secret

Fasting, as a willful act, predates written and spoken history. In humans and other animals fasting is an imprinted wisdom of the natural laws of survival. It has been practiced throughout most, if not all, of our cultural histories, and our religious writings include accounts of Christ, Buddha, Moses, Mohamed, and countless other persons undergoing long water fasts for spiritual as well as physical benefit. Hippocrates, the "father of Western medicine," Socrates, and Plato practiced and advocated fasting,[1] while Pythagoras actually required a forty-day fast of his students as an entrance requirement.[2] Greece, as well as Egypt, Persia, India, and the Gothic and Celtic nations trace their fasting roots to the Ancient Mysteries of early civilization, which also advocated fasting for initiation and therapeutic purposes.[3]

It is widely acknowledged that animals with injury or illness will abstain from food until their health has improved. Most people have personally experienced a loss of appetite with the flu and with viral and bacterial infections as have those people with chronic diseases such as hepatitis, cancer, AIDS, ulcers, colitis, etc. Foods don't taste or smell good, and often nausea, vomiting, or diarrhea accompanies their consumption. We have a natural intuition to fast, animals fast, and our religious and cultural roots are rich in fasting tradition, yet modern medicine has translated this natural law into "eat to keep your strength up." Since natural law does not change, future medicine hopefully will return to this ancient wisdom.

Fasting is not really a secret, but very little information is heard about it because modern medicine is generally critical of and unimpressed by simple noninterventive treatments such as fasting. In the past century people such as Mark Twain, Upton Sinclair, Mahatma Gandhi, and Martin Luther King Jr. wrote about and practiced fasting for health, spiritual, and in Gandhi's case, for protest/penance purposes. While most recognized for his fast to unite India, Gandhi wrote many works on the use of fasting for health including his book *Nature Cure*, published in 1954. Mark Twain wrote in "My Debut as a Literary Person" (1899) that "A little starvation can really do more for the average sick man than can the best medicines and the best doctors." He continues to say from experience, "starvation has been my cold and fever doctor for fifteen years, and has accomplished a cure in all instances."[4]

The word *fast* is derived from the Anglo-Saxon word *faest*, which means firm or fixed. Anytime you fix limitations on the foods that you eat, you are literally fasting. Though the Hygienist[5] practice and many fasting promoters speak of fasting as only that state achieved by complete elimination of all foods (water only), the Catholic practice of meatless Friday is a fast. In fact the Greek Orthodox Church has 181 days per year of restricted diet or fasting. From a medical or therapeutic standpoint the simple elimination of meat or a few foods does not achieve a state of fasting although it does begin the spiritual benefits of willful discipline. To evoke the powerful natural healing of the fast a person has to fix a much more restricted intake of foods. Typically this is accomplished by consuming fresh juices, vegetable broth, and/or water. It is by significantly lightening the physiologic requirements of digestion that the body is able to achieve the remarkable healing powers of fasting.

The Purpose of This Book

The primary purpose of this book is to present fasting as a safe and effective tool for physical, emotional, and spiritual healing. As a therapeutic aid, fasting deserves much more respect and use in modern medicine. Despite its rich history in Western and traditional medicines, fasting lacks the glamour of the "silver bullet" mentality of today's society. It requires a more hands-on relationship between therapist and patient, and it is typically not a high-profit endeavor for either the health care provider or the pharmaceutical industry. The major benefit lies in the health results obtained by the educated faster. It is my belief that science and truth will eventually override the economic drive of modern medicine.

Fasting has been and will continue to be practiced for nontherapeutic reasons. From its earliest practice, fasting has been seen as a discipline of will. Initiation and ceremony will continue to recognize this practice. Fasting has also been used as a form of protest by incarcerated prisoners and by public figures who utilize it to make statements of protest as exemplified by the fasts that Gandhi engaged in for the purpose of peace between Moslem and Hindi people of India. The last time I was in Beijing I spent hours at the Temple of Fasting, where the Chinese emperors of the past would do an annual three-day fast to demonstrate to the people their discipline and sacrifice and to pray for abundant crops.

Fasting also occurs unintentionally when people are trapped or stranded without food. Even though unintentional, these fasts have often accomplished significant improvements in the health of the people involved. Again, Mark Twain wrote much on the health benefits achieved by shipwrecked fasters in the 1800s. Fasting has also served as entertainment in the past, with public exhibits of fasters at world's fairs and other events in the late 1800s and early 1900s in both Europe and America.

Why Fast?

Never in the history of this planet has there been a more important need for the benefits of fasting. We, as humans, have moved farther from the natural environment of the past than at any other time in recorded history. Pollution of air, water, and land is at an all-time high. Our environment is burdened with countless man-made toxins that are measurable in our food and water, and their impact is measurable in our health and diseases. Our foods are less vital, less varied, and highly impactive in the development of cancer, heart disease, and a wide variety of modern illnesses. As we continue to violate natural law and the needs of our species, tools like fasting become critical in our pursuit of quality health.

Detoxification is a major attribute of healthful fasting. Not only does a proper fast enhance the removal of accumulated toxins and wastes, but it also provides an ideal environment for the least damaging removal of the products. The immune system is aided and the liver and kidneys benefit by the reduced demands of normal digestion. The science and physiology of fasting will be discussed in greater detail in the next chapter.

We may choose to fast because of acute or chronic illness or we may choose to fast in pursuit of more radiant health. Fasting has its place as a spiritual practice, as a health maintenance tool, and as a true therapeutic agent.

Concepts of Health

Health is defined in Webster's dictionary as physical, emotional, spiritual, and social well-being.[6] It is a word that's true meaning lies individually within each one of us. For nearly thirty years holistic writers have been talking about health as more than the absence of disease, and to some degree this new concept has become mainstream yet still ambiguous. While the general public is becoming more aware of the concept of optinum health and rediscovering natural therapeutics, the insurance industry and national health care system are actually moving backwards with the creation of HMOs and PPOs which have primarily regulated expenses while de-emphasizing health maintenance and prevention from the holistic paradigm. The "penny wise, pound foolish" mentality of these new systems is being openly challenged by many individuals and groups, yet they remain the "hope for the future" in the words of legislators and lobbyists who promise that with time this broken paradigm will work.

When I was in naturopathic medical school, the concept of health was often presented in the now familiar diagram of the overlap of body, mind, and spirit, with a small overlap of each into a shared tiny area in the center.

While this diagram may have been a necessary first step for a "physical" paradigm of medicine, I believe it to be inaccurate in its exclusion of much greater overlap. In fact I would redraw the circles as one single area with the trilogy of Body, Mind, and Spirit as one common expression of life. I look at physical disease as a more basic communication of illness, often on behalf of the emotions or spirit.

As modern medicine has emerged from the shadows of ignorance and superstition, it has based its present and future on the germ theory of disease. This model has had to broaden itself with the awareness of chronic disease states that abound in current times. Yet, all too frequently, the misguided germ theory paradigm leads modern medicine away from personal responsibility and into the "silver bullet" approach of health care. I use the word "misguided" because the germ theory is traced to Louis Pasteur, and is presented as the trilogy: opportunistic microbe, method of transfer, and susceptible host. Modern medicine has lived on the two-legged stool of antimicrobials and prevention of spread, but has failed miserably to realize Pasteur's wisdom of host or personal susceptibility.

It is time to put the third leg back into this precarious paradigm. We will never have immunizations for every potentially harmful microbe. The list of known pathogens in the bacterial, viral, fungal, and protozoan categories is ever expanding. Some of the most common bacteria have developed resistance to many of our antibiotics, and we have no broadly effective antiviral agents in our modern formulary. We have not been able to provide safe drinking water for the majority of the world's inhabitants, and we are far from a world where all people understand how diseases spread and how through personal hygiene and social awareness we can dramatically reduce the spread of infectious diseases. The preciousness of human life has not been motivation enough to effect a world unity in establishing a healthy planet. Our social, ethnic, national, and class differences pretty much guarantee that infectious disease will not be controlled or eradicated in our lifetimes.

Stress and Disease

Recent human studies have shown that stress, as a single factor, can greatly influence one's susceptibility to infection. In one experiment cited in the *New England Journal of Medicine*, volunteers were exposed singularly to one of three minor respiratory viruses in one of three strengths (titers). The findings consistently showed that how the individuals registered on stress surveys was strongly correlated with the chance of infection and illness. It didn't matter which of the three viruses was used or how strong the dose of the virus was; those people with more stressful life situations were more likely to get sick.[7] Life stress is one of many factors that contribute to your susceptibility to infection or disease.

The concept of stressors as a contributor to disease progression was strongly emphasized in the brilliant work of Hans Seyle, M.D., Ph.D.,

D.Sc. I still consider his textbook *The Physiology and Pathology of Exposure to Stress*, 1950, to be one of my prized possessions. It is a must-read for doctors and health-care providers, especially those who doubt or underplay the significant influence of stress on illness. Seyle provides irrefutable connections between excessive stress (as individually experienced) and cellular, tissue, organ, and indeed whole body damage and disease. He places an importance on nutrition as one of the individual things that can aid in your response to stress, and early on, he recognized that stress is not just a negative event. His definition of a stressor as any event that requires a physiological response by an organism in order to maintain balance or health is still an excellent interpretation.

You cannot and would not want to live in a stress-free environment. Like the "straw that breaks the camel's back," you would like to limit your stress load to a manageable weight and be the strongest camel possible. Stress management involves many different components. How you respond to stress is one important factor, and it starts with recognizing stress and how it influences your daily life. Some personalities appear as stress magnets, and a change of patterns, learning to say no, and reclaiming personal choice in life are a few of the potential solutions found through counseling, personal work, or other methods available. Nutrition is an extremely important factor in how and how well you respond to stress. This is discussed in Chapter 7.

Spiritual Health

Just as the concept of health lacks a precise, quantifiable measurement, the presence or action of the spirit is even more mysterious. There are no gauges to measure the state of the spirit, nor in fact is there any physically measurable entity that science can state is spirit. We can theorize and study the action of prayer on health or disease and you can accept the concept of spirit as a society, in religions, and as individuals, but we are extremely limited in our abilities to assign any measurable property to its presence. This very important element of health is nearly absent in modern medicine and its importance is compromised by its theoretical nature. Traditional medicine, fasting, acupuncture, and Ayurvedic practice are a few of the existing bridges capable of integrating spiritual components into modern practice.

For example, in Ayurvedic tradition, fasting is considered a spiritual practice. First it is indicated for physical concerns including obesity and the condition called "excess *kapha*" (nutritional imbalance). However, because of its positive awakening of the spirit, fasting also is said to be a process of *langhana* or "making one lighter."[8] In a model of health where spirit and body are one, the spiritual changes are inseparable from the physical.

2

The Human Body

The human body is truly remarkable. Throughout every given day systems and cells are processing and integrating more information than any modern computer possibly could. We are only beginning to understand the immense informational network that exists in every cell wall throughout our bodies. While our learning curve has been huge for the past hundred years, there is still so much that remains unknown about how our bodies work, react, and ultimately thrive or expire. Walt Whitman's line from his *Leaves of Grass*, "And a mouse is miracle enough to stagger sextillions of infidels,"[1] is as true today as it was more than a hundred years ago. Life is still the unknown experience.

While we may never understand the full meaning of life or the life processes of the human body, we do know a significant amount about the basic functions such as digestion and elimination of foods and wastes. We are beginning to tie together some of the interactions of various systems of the body, for instance, how stress may negatively affect digestion, immunity, and other normal functions of the healthy individual. We are identifying and naming various chemical messengers within the body's systems and understanding parts of their influence on various activities of cells and tissues. With this added knowledge comes greater power to live life to its fullest.

Normal Anatomy and Physiology of Digestion

If digestion were a mental or cognitive function, we would all be over-whelmed with the labor of eating. Fortunately, the majority of digestion is part of the autonomic nervous system, a self-regulating part of your body that requires no mental or willful action. From the moment you think about food, your digestive system kicks into gear. In fact, 20 percent of your digestive fluids are released in response to the thought, sight, smell, and taste of food.[2] The only intentional components of digestion are the choice and preparation of food, delivery of the food to your mouth, chewing, swallowing, and the final push of waste out the rectum.

As you read through this section on normal digestion, take note of the many organs and cells involved in the breakdown, absorption, and delivery of nutrients throughout the body. Every single component of this process requires energy, oxygen, and blood delivery to the related cells and organs. This is a responsive energy system, relating to the volume and complexity of foods consumed.

Digestion is impacted by a number of extraneous factors; most important is the relative state of stress or adrenaline and cortisol levels at the time of digestion. Other important factors include the cellular health of associated tissues, the bacterial balance of the digestive tract, and the competency of nervous and circulatory systems. This last factor may often include spinal position and integrity but can also include organo-pathologies of the nervous or circulatory systems. While there may be many factors that interfere with optimum digestion, the body efficiently supplies the process of digestion with enough energy to meet the needs of each meal.

The Alimentary Tract

The alimentary tract is the long, multi-shaped tube that runs from the lips and mouth to the rectum and anus. As illustrated in Figure 2.1 on page 12, the alimentary tract begins with the mouth and throat, which share both digestive and respiratory functions. The alimentary tract then continues independently as the esophagus, stomach, small intestine, large intestine, and rectum. This tract, along with support from the kidneys, helps supply and balance the body's water, nutrients, and electrolytes. The liver, gall bladder, and pancreas continue the support of digestion as they release enzymes and bile into the alimentary tract at the level of the small intestine.

Digestion is a process of unified actions within the alimentary tract, coupled with the support of associated organs and systems. There are five major functions that take place during the consumption of food. Food moves through the alimentary tract. There it is mixed with digestive enzymes and is broken down into absorbable particles. Water, electrolytes, and nutrients are absorbed in the small and large intestines. The circulatory system, which supplies the energy needs of digestion, carries the absorbed nutrients to their intermediary and final destinations. The nervous and hormonal systems continuously interact with and support these processes. The movement, digestion, absorption, and delivery actions are almost all controlled by the central nervous system as an autonomic, or nonintentional, process.

Chewing

The first step in normal digestion involves the chewing of solid foods. This process, called mastication, accomplishes three important functions. It reduces the size of your food. It creates a greater surface area for the food's exposure to the enzymes and acids of digestion. It also releases the natural enzymes contained within many foods that aid in their complete digestion.

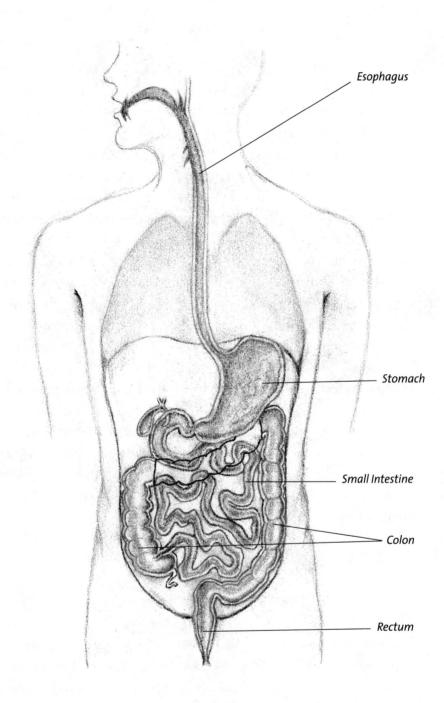

Esophagus

Stomach

Small Intestine

Colon

Rectum

FIGURE 2.1 *The Alimentary Tract*

The act of chewing stimulates the salivary, submandibular, and parotid glands that release their fluids into the mouth. The salivary glands release fluids, which are comprised of water, sodium bicarbonate, potassium, mucus, and ptyalin. As you chew your food, you are mixing the water, electrolytes, and enzymes with each bite. Both the parotid glands and the submandibular glands release the starch-digesting enzyme called ptyalin. This enzyme is identical to the amylase released by the pancreas for the completion of sugar digestion and breakdown in the gut.

According to Guyton and Hall in their *Textbook of Medical Physiology*, up to 40 percent of the digestion of starches can be accomplished prior to delivery of food to the small intestine, the location of the subsequent release of carbohydrate-digesting enzymes by the pancreas. When you don't chew your foods adequately, you are creating a much greater responsibility for the action of the pancreas. Lack of mastication places us at risk for incomplete digestion of starches, thereby supplying your body with less available energy and opening the door for other detrimental consequences. The mucus, or mucoid proteins, released by the glands of the mouth help provide lubrication and protection to the mucus membranes of the throat and esophagus during the passage of chewed material.

The actions of the glands of the mouth and the digestive system as a whole are influenced by the senses of sight, smell, and taste. The olfactory glands, which are responsible for the sense of smell, are neurochemically involved in releasing digestive fluids and in stimulating the gut-associated immune function. All three of the sense organs contribute to and impact upon normal digestion.

Swallowing and the Gastroesophageal Sphincter Valve

The act of swallowing propels food down the esophagus, which connects the throat and mouth with the stomach. Swallowing triggers a relaxation of the cardiac sphincter, recently renamed the gastroesophageal sphincter, the valve that lets food into the stomach but prevents the return of food or stomach acids back up the esophagus. If this sphincter is inflamed, scarred, or in spasm, the common symptoms of heartburn or more severe esophageal reflux conditions can occur.

The Stomach

The stomach has a number of important functions. It stores the majority of your food as it slowly allows small portions into the small intestine for further digestion. The stomach also has cells that communicate with the central nervous system and cells that release important materials such as HCl (hydrochloric acid), the substance required for the conversion of secreted pepsinogen into its protein-digesting form, called pepsin. Cells in the stomach also release a substance called intrinsic factor that is required for the absorption of vitamin B_{12}. Since stomach acid is an essential component of protein digestion and of the activation of the protein breakdown enzyme pepsin, the use of antacids for heartburn alters the stomach's intended acid environment for optimal digestion of proteins. There are much better ways to get adequate dietary calcium than through the use of calcium carbonate supplements, which also reduce the absorption of calcium since stomach acid is required for the absorption of some minerals including calcium.

The Pyloric Sphincter Valve

As foods and fluids continue to pass through the alimentary canal they come to a complete valve at the end of the stomach. This valve, called the pyloric sphincter, is regulated by the vagal nerve through its influence on the actions of the stomach. It is this valve that regulates the release of foods into the small intestine, where digestion is completed and absorption begins. The pyloric sphincter is considered a complete valve since food is never allowed to reenter the stomach through this structure. On the other hand, the gastroesophageal sphincter is an incomplete valve because it allows reverse emptying of the stomach, which is commonly called vomiting. Vomiting is a necessary and logical process that allows us to expel poisonous or contaminated foods that may have been ingested.

The Small Intestine

The small intestine, which averages about fifteen feet in length, is divided into three regions named the duodenum, the jejunum, and the ileum. There are physical, cellular, and functional differences between each of these three regions. The duodenum, which is connected to the stomach, receives the partially digested foods from the stomach and mixes them with a broad array of fat-, starch-, and protein-digesting enzymes provided by the pancreas. These pancreatic enzymes enter the duodenum with bile from the liver and gall bladder through an opening called the hepatopancreatic ampulla. In most people the gall bladder releases bile into a duct, or tube, that joins with the hepatic duct of the liver becoming the common hepatic duct. This duct in turn connects with the pancreatic duct to create a common duct through which the mixture of fluids is released into the duodenum.

As mentioned earlier, starches are ideally predigested with the aid of the glandular enzymes supplied in the mouth and through the actions of the stomach secretions. Proteins are partially digested in the stomach, and fats are basically held unchanged until their release into the small intestine. The many enzymes released by the pancreas are responsible for the complete and final digestion of starches and sugars, for the breakdown of fats into absorbable molecules, and for the reduction of proteins to the smallest peptide forms necessary for absorption. Cells within the intestinal tract are responsible for cleaving these peptides into the individual amino acids that are the building-block forms of the proteins required for human life.

Some polysaccharides, or complex starches, as well as hormone-like proteins can be absorbed intact, but most foods must be broken down to their most simple nutritional structures for optimum absorption to take place. Most nutrients are absorbed in the jejunum and the ileum. Nearly all fat and bile re-uptake takes place in the ileum. Electrolytes and water are absorbed in the small intestine, but the final uptake and balancing of electrolytes and fluids takes place in the large intestine.

Bile is the soap of the human digestive system. It is produced in the liver as a combination of bile salts, cholesterol, and lecithin. When released into the small intestine it helps to emulsify fat molecules. Emulsification allows fats to be suspended in the salt-water-based bloodstream of humans, much like dish detergent allows fats to be suspended in dishwater. You reabsorb 90 to 95 percent of your bile in the ileum, and once the fats are removed from it, the bile is conjugated, or preserved, by the liver for storage in the gall bladder. Bile is what gives feces their brown coloring. The more fiber you have in your diet, the more bile is eliminated with your stool as opposed to being reabsorbed. This is the primary link between dietary fiber and lowered cholesterol levels in humans. Since bile is primarily composed of cholesterol, its elimination helps to lower your levels of circulating cholesterol.

With the release of fluids from the cells of the mouth, esophagus, stomach, small intestine, liver, gall bladder, and pancreas, you process your food in a highly liquid form. This is important to allow the maximum contact between enzymes and the food particles. Once the digestive breakdown of foods is complete, it is important to conserve the precious fluids of the body. The large intestine serves to dehydrate the liquid wastes as well as reabsorb important electrolytes. The tissues of the colon are a two-way dynamic structure, able to regulate fluids, to secrete mucus, and, through lymphatic secretory canals, to eliminate toxic products circulating through the lymph system. For example, heavy metals like cadmium and mercury can be dumped into the large intestine and eliminated with the dietary wastes via these lymphatic structures.

The Ileocecal Valve

The ileum of the small intestine connects with the colon at what is called the ileocecal valve. This incomplete valve is located in the lower right region of the abdomen, where the appendix is typically located. The large intestine ascends up the abdomen, toward the liver, crosses, or transverses, the abdomen and descends down the left side where it ends as the rectum (see Figure 2.2). The rectum is the temporary storage area for these processed wastes until nature calls for a bowel movement.

When foods, water, and electrolytes are absorbed, they are carried in the bloodstream to the liver and other areas of the body. Storage, conversion, and utilization of these nutrients are needed to complete the digestive process.

Digestion Is Work

As you have seen, there is a great deal of activity and work being performed every time food is consumed. Your body has the ability to do this work for every meal, every day of your life. The more energy needed for impaired health and stress management, the harder it is to digest and utilize foods to their greatest benefit. When you fast on fresh vegetable juices that are almost self-digesting, you are sparing your entire body from a great deal of daily labor. This increase in available energy is used for other important repair and maintenance processes.

Cellular and Neurologic Control of Digestion

In the previous section I presented a very brief overview of how food passes through the alimentary tract and some information on the digestion and absorption of nutrients. While I included comments on the great amount of cellular and systemic energy that is required for effective use of foods, the complete energy of digestion includes additional factors.

There is an extensive process of cellular and neurologic communication that takes place with every meal. Cells within the mouth, nose, stomach, and small intestine report to the brain and associated glands about the composition of what has been consumed. The brain interprets this information and communicates to the various digestive structures so that

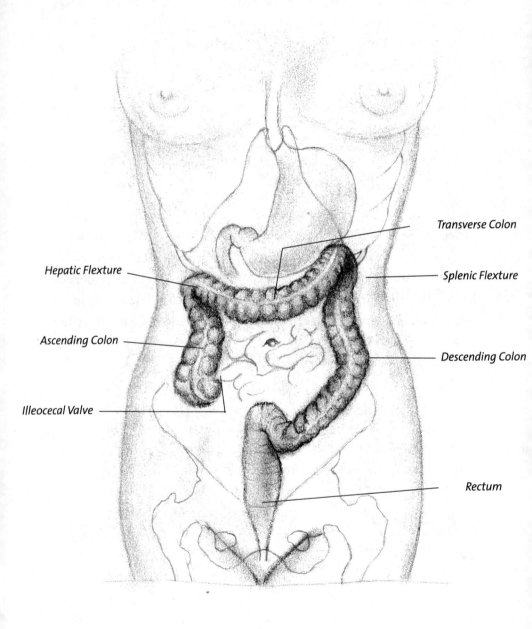

FIGURE 2.2 *The Large Intestine*

they respond appropriately for the optimum breakdown and absorption of your foods. Some of this is mediated directly through the cranial nerves, particularly the optic, olfactory, and vagal nerves. These nerves, originating from the brain stem, are responsible for many of the normal functions of the digestive system. The functional component of the nervous system that is responsible for normal digestion is called the parasympathetic nervous system. This system can be inhibited by the sympathetic nervous system, often called the "fight or flight" system. The sympathetic system is closely associated with adrenal function and the presence or absence of adrenaline and cortisol in the bloodstream.

When you are alarmed, frightened, or extremely stressed you release adrenaline into the bloodstream. Adrenaline can be a lifesaving chemical when it makes you stronger or faster so you can avoid or confront imminent danger. Part of this strength comes from the action of adrenaline pushing more sugar into cells, but a large part of the additional strength and energy comes from the changes of blood flow and delivery that accompany higher adrenaline levels. The human body is wise enough to know that when you are running from a bear or enemy you should not be investing your energy and oxygen into digestive processes. During sympathetic activity, blood is diverted from digestion, immune function, and skin to deliver additional blood to the brain and muscles. This is important on a short-term basis, but chronic stress can lead to significant disturbances in digestive and immune functions.

Cortisol is an important hormone released by the adrenal cortex. Its functions include control of the metabolism of proteins, carbohydrates, and fats. It also aids in the body's ability to control inflammatory processes and helps to offset excessive adrenal response to stress. There are nutritional factors that are associated with the normal production of cortisol as well as an association with both light (sun) stimulation and the presence of an internally produced pre-hormone called DHEA. Exercise also enhances cortisol balance.

Chronic excessive stress requires higher levels of cortisol and so digestion is often incomplete, which can lead to more microbial overgrowth in the gut as well as the development of food sensitivities. Chronically impaired or reduced circulation to the digestive system due to increased sympathetic stimulation can also affect the normal repair and replacement processes of digestive tissues and structures. This can, in turn, exacerbate a number of digestive diseases like esophageal reflux, irritable bowel syndrome, and colitis. Normalization of the digestive system may often require reducing stress or managing stress more effectively, thereby reducing sympathetic stimulation. Fasting can be one tool to help reverse the negative influences of chronic stress. Other aids can include the B vitamins, vitamins C and E, aerobic exercise, deep breathing, biofeedback, or various counseling techniques. The avoidance of stimulants, especially caffeine, can also help manage excessive stress.

When the sympathetic system is not overriding the normal parasympathetic control of digestion, there is a very efficient cooperation between the digestive system and the brain. You absorb nutrients both in the mouth and aromatically by the olfactory glands of the nose. These initial food products, when perceived by the brain, stimulate the release of saliva and digestive enzymes, as well as help initiate the proper environment for complete digestion of foods.

As food enters the stomach, another feedback loop begins between the digestive system and the brain. A number of changes occur within the digestive feedback loops. Some foods are absorbed and communicate the anticipated needs of stomach and pancreatic secretions regarding the appropriate digestion of fat, protein, and sugars. The stretching of the cells of the stomach lining activates another important feedback loop. When the stomach is stretched there is a release of a chemical called gastrin, stimulating the release of hydrochloric acid, which is essential in the conversion of pepsinogen into pepsin, an active protein-digesting enzyme. Pepsinogen is an inactive chemical that is released in response to hydrochloric acid release and in response to vagal stimulation from neurologic feedback. If you have inadequate levels of hydrochloric acid in the stomach (from taking antacids), you cannot adequately convert pepsinogen into its active pepsin form and that can cause protein digestion to be impaired.

Vagal and chemical feedback continue throughout the intestinal tract. This information helps to establish the ideal environment throughout the digestive tract for optimum utilization of your nutrients. The pancreas is responsible for the majority of digestive breakdown of your foods. The pancreas creates protein-digesting enzymes, amino acidases, RNA- and DNA-ases, and other protease enzymes that are essential in the reduction of proteins to the small peptide molecules necessary for absorption in the small intestine. The pancreas is also responsible for the reduction of fats into absorbable nutrients and for the reduction of starches into the desired six-carbon simple sugars, such as glucose, which provide the most abundant fuel and energy source for the human system.

This has again been a very brief overview of the complex and high-energy functions of digestion and absorption. My favorite source of current information on digestion is the medical text used by most medical colleges called *Textbook of Medical Physiology*, by Guyton and Hall. It is very extensive and has been respected for decades as one of the most authoritative and accurate texts of its kind. My overview has primarily served to help you understand the significant reduction of energy requirements that accompanies a fasting program. It is certainly not necessary to be an authority on the physiology of digestion to benefit from the digestive changes and rest accomplished by a juice fast.

Normal Elimination and Removal of Toxins

Just as you have a constant need for water, electrolytes, and nutrients, you have a constant need to eliminate the indigestible portions of your foods, the wastes of cellular actions, and the by-products of cellular breakdown and death. If you were not in a steady state of elimination of these wastes, you would grow to thousands of pounds by the time you reached mid-life. You would not live in a home; you would just drape a big circus tent over your immense body with a few openings for interacting with the outside world. This seems like an absurd discussion but is ironically a relevant point that is missed by the many skeptics of the benefits of fasting.

Every living cell in your body has eliminatory requirements and actions. These actions are typically normal metabolic features of each cell, although they can be influenced by both external and internal factors. Nutrition, both good and bad, environmental toxins and chemicals, as well as prescription and nonprescription drugs can increase or decrease individual elimination pathways of your cells. Your own physiologic environment (hormones, circulation, and other neurochemical mediators) can also dramatically influence the functioning of your cells. Nutritional and physiologic balance in cellular health and metabolism is one of the starting points of functional eliminatory processes.

There are many organs and systems involved with the elimination of wastes. These include the lungs, the skin and mucus tissues, the kidneys, the liver, the spleen, the intestines, and the immune system. (See Figure 2.3.) Most of the eliminatory processes are basic and straightforward; however there are unique properties associated with both the liver and the immune system that deserve special attention. These will be discussed in Chapter 5 as normal autolysis and elimination are compared to the enhanced state of detoxification achieved in fasting.

The Lungs

The lungs are the most essential, most active, and most productive eliminatory organs of the body. Their elimination of carbon dioxide in exchange with oxygen must be maintained on a continual basis or death will occur rapidly. The primary function of your lungs is to absorb oxygen as O_2 through tissue linings and to eliminate carbon dioxide (CO_2) through these same tissues. Secondary functions include removal of noxious products and other volatile chemicals as well as the elimination of physical matter through the expectoration of mucus.

When you inhale you are not taking in pure oxygen. The air you breathe is comprised of a number of chemicals including nitrogen, car-

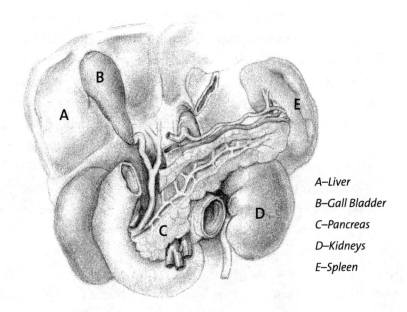

A–Liver
B–Gall Bladder
C–Pancreas
D–Kidneys
E–Spleen

FIGURE 2.3 *Organs of Digestion and Elimination*

bon dioxide, and a vast array of airborne substances. These substances include:

- Bacteria
- Viruses
- Spores from fungi
- Pollens, dust
- Natural and manmade chemicals including carbon monoxide, sulfur compounds
- Petrochemical fumes and by-products

Your body knows to return the carbon dioxide and nitrogen to the outside air, but many of the other chemicals, especially fat-loving, or lipophilic, chemicals are either absorbed into the bloodstream or remain in the tissues of the lungs. When you inspire chemicals into your bloodstream, they can either be expired out of your system or they can be eliminated through other systems. If you are breathing in noxious fumes, you will not eliminate more than you absorb until you receive fresher air. As global air quality continues to decline, the use of a home air filter becomes more practical and necessary. We may find a need for supplemental oxygen in our environment as the oxygen content of the air continues its alarming decline. The emergence of "oxygen bars" is a visible first step in that direction.

When you respire substances into the tissues of your lungs, there are many adaptive responses. You have small hairs, or cilia, that help move mucus, fluids, and material up the lungs and eventually out of the body. For microbes like viruses and bacteria and for small peptides such as pollens, the removal is assisted by the action of the white blood cells as they work to destroy these invaders. Some foreign substances, which are not easily removed, remain for long periods in the lungs. Tars from tobacco can stain and remain in the tissues for the life of a chronic smoker. Asbestos will be encapsulated, like a pearl,[3] in tissues where it remains. Fortunately most foreign substances either pass through, are reduced by immune action, or are expectorated by the mechanical action of the lungs.

Deep breathing and exercise are helpful in the overall eliminatory functions of the lungs. The fasting physiology is also very helpful for these processes. There is a consistent reduction in the thickness and quantity of mucus in people who are fasting. There is also a reduction in allergic influence and an enhanced immune response. Often people who are fasting will experience an increase in expectoration and elimination from the lungs. This is a normal and healthy process associated with the detoxification of fasting.

Most fasts, including the fasting diet, will also greatly enhance the sense of smell. Both pleasant and unpleasant odors will be magnified by the typical changes of the fasting physiology. Olfactory response (the neurologic recognition of odors) is known to help or hinder both digestion and immune function. Walks in the outdoors (beaches, woods, and the like—not freeways and industrial sites) provide some wonderful support for these olfactory responses. Whole foods will also reveal their pleasant flavors and aromas in an enhanced manner upon reintroduction to your solid diet.

The Kidneys

The kidneys are a sophisticated filtration system, filtering more than 180 liters of blood per day. They filter out microscopic wastes from the bloodstream and reabsorb important electrolytes to help regulate the fluid balance of your entire body. Their filtration processes can be compared to a colander you use to rinse off foods. The holes in your kidney filters are too small for red blood cells, white blood cells, proteins, and other larger structures to pass through. Minerals and some heavy metals can easily pass through this filter, but mercury is reported to be impassable. When wastes are too big to eliminate through the kidneys, they can be eliminated through a different organ, modified chemically for removal, or stored in the body.

While the kidney has a functional wisdom that retains important electrolytes, its function is highly dependent upon your intake of water and other hydrating fluids. Just as you could not rinse off a cup of berries with a teaspoon of water, your kidneys cannot adequately carry out chemical wastes with inadequate hydration. The carrying capacity of water is called its solubility coefficient or in medical considerations, the specific gravity, which is a measure of the amount of substance currently in solution. Most people have gargled with salt-water for a sore throat or shared in the experience of watching as you add salt to water. Initially the salt is contained in solution, but as you continue to add salt it settles, or precipitates, to the bottom of the glass. This is the same principle that influences your ability to eliminate wastes through the kidneys. If you have inadequate fluid, similar to the salt settling to the bottom of the glass, the wastes are left behind, settling in your body's tissues.

Over the years I have performed thousands of urine evaluations on my fasting participants. This test is commonly called a chemical urinalysis. With simple indicator strips we can measure a number of urine wastes and contents. The strips I use include specific gravity, pH, glucose, and ketones. I perform these tests prior to the fast, during the pre-fast diet, and on the third day of the juice phase. A pattern is clearly visible when comparing these three samples. Initially people will have a high specific gravity and a low pH, indicating high acidity. These numbers would improve during the pre-fast and typically become both alkaline and much more dilute during the final phase.

These are very important changes when it comes to optimum elimination of wastes. The human measurement of specific gravity has a range of 1.000 to 1.030. With 1.000 defined as the standard weight of distilled water, 1.030 is the heaviest that water can attain while carrying foreign materials. Most of the pre-fast urines were 1.025–1.030, meaning that there was little or no room left to carry out additional wastes. During the juice phase the specific gravity would average 1.005–1.010, and not surprisingly, with a more dilute urine the acids of normal elimination were much more dilute, and the urine ranged from slightly acidic to slightly alkaline or basic.

Water is one of the most overlooked and important medicines of any time. When you are dehydrated many negative consequences result. Low energy, fatigue, or even depression can accompany inadequate fluid intake. Many physical health consequences can occur with poor fluid intake. These physical impacts will occur throughout the body in nearly every organ and system. I always wonder how much of the benefit that people attribute to natural products and prescription drugs is associated with the improved hydration from the water required to swallow the pills!

The easiest way I have found to explain specific gravity and hydration to my patients is with the following analogy. Consider water to be a bus with thirty seats. This bus tours throughout your body picking up passengers with some degree of preferential treatment for the loud and obnoxious passengers like nitrogen and ammonia from protein metabolism. Once the bus is full, no more commuters get picked up at the bus stops. Hopefully a new bus will soon be by with empty seats. The longer the commuters wait, the more irritable they become.

Many people think that any fluid they drink has thirty available seats. This is far from true. Some fluids, like those high in sugar, such as juice, soda pop, and milk, come into our bodies with their seats already taken. Other fluids with chemicals called diuretics, like coffee or caffeine products, speed through like an empty bus that doesn't stop for passengers. Some products like alcohol, which is both high in sugar and a diuretic, can actually dehydrate the body with excessive consumption. For the purposes of hydration, water, noncaffeine tea, and diluted juice are the beverages of choice.

The body is aware of the need to remove highly inflammatory substances like nitrogen and ammonia, so it will donate fluid from one system to another in order to reduce inflammation. The most abundant source of fluid is found in the colon. When the kidneys require reserve sources of fluid it is not uncommon to see constipation follow. With less fluid available to the colon, the skin is called to additional action and "eliminatory rashes" are not uncommon. As a rule you should like to see your urine maintain a clear to slightly yellow appearance. If your urine is regularly dark yellow to orange, you need to increase the intake of helpful fluids. The vitamin riboflavin will color your urine bright yellow even with good hydration. Do not consider this visible show of yellow following the intake of B vitamins to be an indicator of inadequate hydration.

Highly acid urine (pH 5.0) is often an indicator of the bus seats being full. Many of the normal cellular and nutritional functions of the body release acids into the bloodstream; therefore the urine pH is a valuable indicator of hydration. Your tissues and body have a safe range of acidity and alkalinity that they must maintain. If you exceed this range in either direction, tissue damage and other serious consequences will occur. Intake of oxygen helps to regulate the pH balance, with increased oxygen resulting in decreased acidity. Most Americans maintain an acid environment that borders on the upper end of the range. High-acid-producing foods like wheat, meat, sugar, and coffee have offset the historical alkalinizing influence of vegetables and the less-acidic cereals and grains. Inadequate water only compounds this problem.

The Skin and Mucus Tissues

The skin and mucus tissues of the body have many functions that are essential to quality of life. Your skin, the tissues that surround your body, serves primarily to protect you from outside or environmental insult including dehydration, mechanical trauma, and infection. It is a major sensory organ helping you accommodate to temperature variations and to other environmental information. It is the location of ultraviolet conversion of provitamin D into the vitamin's active form.

The skin is structurally distinct from internal mucus linings or tissues. One of these differences is the nearly waterproof surface of your skin, which is comprised of keratin. The keratin, a protective protein, of the outer skin ranges from an extremely thin layer in the soft regions of the abdomen, wrist, neck, etc., to much thicker regions such as the palms of the hands and soles of the feet. The skin also is strongly attached to underlying connective tissues that help in motion and in protection against detachment.

What makes the skin a part of the normal eliminatory system is the presence of sweat and oil glands that are part of normal skin structure. The sweat glands are primarily used by the body to help regulate temperature, but they also eliminate electrolytes, fluids, and other minerals during the heat-regulatory process. The oil glands, called sebaceous glands, are a much more important part of the skin's eliminatory functions.

The sebaceous glands are found in most parts of the skin but are absent in the palms of the hands and soles of the feet. They are most abundant in the scalp and face and are also found in greater abundance around the mouth, anus, ears, and nose as well as under the arms and in the tissues of the chest and upper back. They are important lubricators of your skin and can also serve to eliminate fat-soluble and mineral-based toxins. When your internal eliminatory functions are incomplete, the skin is called upon to assist the maintenance of a healthy environment. These processes can be enhanced by nutritional and physical supports, such as saunas and hydrotherapy.

The skin has associated glands, called follicles and beds, which make hair and nails respectively. As skin sloughs off dead cells and hair and nails are removed, there are measurable toxic wastes that are being returned to the outside environment. Heavy metals and other environmental toxins can be chemically isolated and measured from samples of hair, nails, and skin.

The skin and internal mucus tissues are significantly influenced by adrenal response to stress. As you release adrenaline in a fear response, it significantly alters the flow of blood to these tissues. Stress is a highly functional response that puts most of circulatory function and energy into the muscles and brain so you can escape a perceived threat to live another day. Chronic stress will lead to chronic digestive and skin-related conditions, due to decreased blood flow and waste removal and other hormone-related factors. It is no coincidence that you get a pimple before an important date or see your skin's appearance worsen during high stress periods of life.

The mucus tissues line the body's air pathways, alimentary canal, vagina, and urinary system. Each of these regions has its own specific functional requirements, and its physical structures are related to these needs. While the mucus tissues are protective and absorptive in nature, they are also eliminatory and waste-secreting structures. Not only can individual cells release wastes, but within some mucus tissues, lymph canals drain directly into the gastrointestinal (GI) tract for elimination.

Historically, humans had a diet that was much more abundant in fiber, essential fats, beta-carotene, and other nutrients that support optimum health for your skin and mucus tissues. Our ancestors had a much less toxic environment from the standpoint both of air and of food. As our lifestyles and dietary habits have changed, the secondary or additional responsibility of waste removal by the skin and mucus tissues has increased. In my many years of treating people, I have found that the vast majority of skin conditions like eczema, psoriasis, and seborrhea are directly related to digestive absorption and poor eliminatory function.

The Large Intestine

The digestive system, with its alimentary canal, has the primary responsibility of absorbing nutrients and water from your diet while eliminating or disposing of the indigestible components of your foods. In addition to indigestible fibers and nonutilized food-related compounds, your digestive waste includes significant living and dead bacteria that are necessary features of a healthy digestive system. The importance and purpose of these friendly microbes will be discussed in detail in the next section.

As the alimentary canal transitions from the small intestine to the large intestine, digestion and absorption of food-related nutrients are nearly complete. The large intestine still absorbs significant water and electrolytes but primarily acts to push the waste materials to the rectum for final elimination. Eliminated feces are about one-fourth solid and three-fourths water. The solid matter is made up of one-third dead bacteria, one-third fiber and roughage, and the remainder of fat, inorganic matter, and lesser amounts of protein and sloughed or dead cell wastes of normal digestive function.[4]

The large intestine is normally an absorptive organ, taking in as much as five to seven liters of fluid per day. When the large intestine is inflamed or infection is present, it can become an excretory structure, losing up to ten liters of fluid per day. These fluids are both from dietary sources as well as the digestive fluids and secretions from your own cells. The absorption of fluids in the colon is strongly related to both dietary hydration and dietary fiber. The muscles of the large intestine need wastes to be firm enough to push, but soft enough to pass. Constipation is a common response to inadequate fiber or fluid in your diet.

The composition of normal feces mentioned above is a list of what is left from the consumption of a "typical" diet. The typical diet of today is far from a colon-friendly diet. I would expect that the composition of feces in earlier times would have had a much higher fiber component and different fat and inorganic constituents. In J. H. Kellogg's book *Colon Hygiene*, in which he emphasized a high-fiber fruit and vegetable diet, he maintained that three bowel movements a day with rapid total transit (elimination of a day's food the same day or the next day) was an ideal norm. For the contemporary or modern American diet, this frequency would only represent an inflammatory or stress-related process. I believe that with an optimum diet (much more fiber—fresh vegetables and other whole foods), three bowel movements a day is not an unhealthy pattern.

Two other eliminatory processes are occurring within the large intestine. In its walls are direct lymph canal pathways. Your body is able to eliminate substances from the bloodstream and regional lymph system directly into the large intestine. This method allows these substances to bypass the liver and the kidney and pass out of your body with normal elimination. There are many things that can assist this pathway, the most basic being fluid and fiber.

Another product being eliminated by the large intestine is what is called xenobiotic wastes. These are the chemicals that are introduced through food and the environment as well as produced in the life processes of the various bacteria and microbes that inhabit the intestinal tract. Microbial by-products are recognized as a significant portion of fecal fat content, but they can be quite varied, dependant on types and populations of microbes as well as dietary habits. The consumed xenobiotic chemicals include pesticides, hormones in meat and dairy, drugs and so-called inert ingredients of many products, and chemicals delivered via the air into the lungs or through the mucus tissues of the respiratory system. The reabsorption of these chemicals in both the small and large intestines can have significant impact on your health. This issue is a central theme of this chapter's section on dysbiosis.

The Immune System and Liver

All six major areas of elimination interact with and depend on the functional integrity of the others. The liver and immune system are alike in these cooperative relationships but also share a greater interdependency. The liver produces immune chemicals and is supportive in the immune process of reducing toxins to a form that can be eliminated. They are uniquely alike in that both white blood cells and the liver can create new metabolic pathways for the reduction of man-made, never-before-encountered chemicals. When you depart from natural and normal elimination of wastes and toxins to the real-world eliminatory needs of modern times, it is the liver and immune system that creatively respond to these needs.

The immune system includes white blood cells, the thymus gland, the spleen, bone marrow, the liver, lymph nodes and lymph canals throughout the body, and numerous lymph structures of the intestinal tract. Your white blood cells are not only responsible for fighting off infectious microbes but also mediate inflammation and the removal of cellular wastes and dead or cancerous cells from your entire body.

The removal of cellular waste and debris can be accomplished by a number of processes. White blood cells can ingest materials and process them internally. They can release immunoglobulins to break up the debris in the fluids of the body, or they can migrate into lymph nodes where a concerted, chemically mediated reduction occurs. Fluids mixed with waste travel via lymph canals to the bloodstream where they can be further reduced by the white pulp of the spleen or by the liver. These modified wastes are released back into the bloodstream where they may be eliminated by any of the major eliminatory systems.

Books are written on the role of the liver in removing wastes. The liver is constantly breaking down molecules into either usable or removable forms. It is in the liver where most of the metabolism and clearing of pharmaceutical drugs takes place. It is also in the liver that most of the normal breakdown of most consumed and internally created toxins occurs. The liver never directly eliminates toxins, but modifies them into forms that can be eliminated by other pathways.

Mitochondria are structures found within human, animal, and plant cells. They are especially concentrated in the cells of the liver and are major sources of both energy production and toxin removal. Within the mitochondria are found numerous chemicals called cytochromes, which have been identified as the major chemical-reducing agents of drugs and other organo-chemicals. There are many different classes and forms of these cytochrome agents including the most widely studied form called cytochrome 450. It is clear from contemporary research that different cytochromes are used for different detoxification pathways. Much like a golfer uses different clubs depending upon the need of each stroke, the body knows which pathway to utilize based upon the structure of the drugs or toxins it encounters. Unlike the golf bag, the human body has hundreds to thousands of combination pathways to choose from.

While the cytochrome pathways are major participants in detoxification, there are many supportive and alternative routes of chemical modification and removal. One of the most important secondary pathways involves the naturally produced chemical glutathione. The glutathione pathways are essential minor players in the complete modification of most drugs. These pathways can be depleted or exhausted when the body's glutathione reserves are used up because of nutritional inadequacy and excessive detoxification demand. That often leads to accumulation of toxic substances in your tissues and cells. Vitamin E, vitamin C, and selenium are significant players in the glutathione reductase activity of human detoxification. While the USDA and FDA do not measure glutathione content in foods, it is logical that all plant mitochondria would possess glutathione as well as other cytochrome structures that can serve as micronutrients in your foods. Vegetable juices would serve as one of the highest sources of plant-based nutrition.

There has been more contemporary research into the removal or clearance of wastes by the liver than by any of the other eliminatory systems. Many individual eliminatory pathways of the liver have been iden-

tified and researched. Drug interactions, drug toxicity, and chemical toxicity are some of the major reasons that these pathways are under
increased study. The general maintenance of health can benefit from this
new knowledge, but one or more of these individual pathways can never
represent the overall and complete function of the liver. We are far from
a complete understanding of the complete works of the liver. Traditional
medicine incorporated a much greater respect for the eliminatory functions of the liver than does our current model. There is wisdom in our
traditions, which can still serve us today.

The Fasting Diet Aids Elimination

The internal environment created by the fasting diet is supportive of all
these major eliminatory processes. Some of the most vocal critics of fasting state that fasting does not increase the elimination of toxins from your
body, but this point of view is not substantiated by either logical arguments or clinical evidence. Dr. Paul Bragg was famous for his chemical
assays of urine and feces during fasts, and he frequently reported high
concentrations of heavy metals, pesticides, and other toxic chemicals.

If you were eating an entirely organic and historically balanced diet,
you would probably be keeping up with your normal eliminatory needs.
Most Americans today manifest the presence of toxins in their tissues
and fat cells, and most people are far from optimally efficient in their
eliminatory processes. The high-fiber and high-fluid content of the pre-
fast diet and the high-nutrition and high-fluid content of the juice phase
significantly reduce normal eliminatory requirements while increasing
normal elimination.

Microflora Out of Balance: Intestinal Dysbiosis

Intestinal dysbiosis is one of the most important and widespread iatrogenic diseases of the twentieth century. The term *iatrogenic* literally

means "produced by physician"[5] and today refers to any harm that results from treatment, misdiagnosis, or side effects of drugs used in medicine. While dysbiosis is endemic in modern society, conventional medicine remains unaware or in denial of its actual existence. Since this disease is primarily caused by the accepted practices of medicine and agriculture, we are far from acknowledging its widespread impact.

Intestinal dysbiosis is a self-descriptive term that means "wrong life in the intestines" and refers to the presence and overgrowth of opportunistic and pathogenic microbes. The overuse and misuse of antibiotics and steroids in both medicine and agriculture create this overgrowth. It is a recent human problem that dates back to the 1940s but has progressively worsened since that time. It is inclusive of the condition termed "systemic Candidiasis" and is considerably varied in its many individual presentations.

The earliest roots of dysbiosis go back to the work of Pasteur and the development of the germ theory. As doctors and scientists looked for microbial or germ causes for disease, they came to understand that there were both beneficial microbes and disease-causing, or pathogenic, microbes. Loudon Douglas, F.R.S.E, in his 1911 book *The Bacillus of Long Life*, recognized and identified dozens of friendly bacteria associated with the many cultured dairy beverages of traditional diets around the world, such as the Armenian soured milk "matzoon," the Greek curdled milk "giaourti," Bulgarian "yoghoort" milk, the Indian soured milk "dadhi," the soured milk "kefir," and buttermilk. Mr. Douglas put forth the proposition that these cultured beverages had significant health benefits associated with their use. We now understand that these benefits are both from the improved digestibility, or bioavailability, due to the partial predigestion of the dairy products by these organisms and from the overall support or reseeding of friendly intestinal flora.

Antibiotics

In 1929 Professor Alexander Fleming discovered that a fungus from the *Penicillium* family produced a chemical that destroyed living bacteria in his laboratory cultures. He coined the name *penicillin* in 1929[6] as the first antibiotic produced by a living organism. His discovery was noted in the medical literature but remained undeveloped until the onset of the Second World War necessitated the rapid development of antibiotics. With the dramatic need came significant research and development in the area of antibiotic medicine. The soil was recognized as a potent source of possible antibiotic-producing organisms, and the identification and isolation of these organisms led to the development of erythromycin, tetracycline, and a host of related antimicrobials.

Medical science investigated possible new sources of antibiotics while refining the methods of cultivating, or growing, the *Penicillium* fungi and improving extraction techniques. This was an important part of the development of current antibiotics, but the original fungi did not produce the amount, or yield, of penicillin desired for medical purposes. In 1940 the original, natural strains of *Penicillium* were exposed both to irradiation and later to damaging ultraviolet light resulting in a mutated form of *Penicillium* that produced huge amounts of penicillin.[7] This form of genetic manipulation, though crude, was the precursor to the more sophisticated genetic modification of today's food supply.

Microbes in Our Soils

The fact that there are fungi in our soils that produce antibiotic chemicals is not an accident or coincidence. We find the source of some of our most potent antifungal agents from soil bacteria. This is because bacteria and fungi share and compete with each other in our planet's organic resources. This is an essential living process that produces the fertile soils from which plant life can grow and thrive. Without the actions of bacteria and fungi, the organic wastes of plant and animal life would not undergo adequate decomposition to build our needed soil.

The bacteria and fungi of the soil are looking after their own life needs; they would both like to have access to as much decomposing organic matter as possible. Like animals that compete for the same food source, these microbes have a bark and a bite that can help defend their food supply. These are mainly chemicals they release to keep their competitors from consuming their desired meals. We call these chemicals antibiotics and antifungals. In the world of the soil, it takes very little antibiotic to chase away the competition; in the systemic world of animals, it takes unusually huge concentrations of antibiotics to battle pathogenic bacteria. The friendly human bacteria have about as much hope of surviving these antibiotic doses as a normal deer would have being hunted by a thousand-foot-tall lion (proportionate to the increase in concentration of antibiotics from medically altered growth and extraction technology).

Microbes in Our Bodies

In healthy humans there exist trillions of "friendly" microbes that assist digestion and help defend against infection. These friendly microbes, which include *Lactobacillus acidophilus*, not only are essential components of digestion and absorption, but their populations occupy and colonize regions that would otherwise support the growth of harmful organisms. A good analogy of this phenomenon is the farming use of cover crops such as clover and vetch that are planted after harvest to prevent the growth of weeds, which steal nutrients from the soil and prohibit the planting of new crops. An even better analogy is an old self-sustaining forest that has never been harvested. The soil that is needed for weeds and nonindigenous plants is always occupied by native vegetation. For this reason, invasion and overgrowth by nonnative plants rarely occurs in a healthy forest.

Human Soil Consumption

There is a logical and important relationship that exists between the normal microbes of the soil and the normal friendly flora of the intestinal tract. While there can be harmful or pathological microbes in the soil, the common soil bacteria include such well-known species as *Lactobacillus acidophilus* and *Bifidobacterium bifidum* as well as many other friendly bacteria. As our ancestors consumed soil residues in their foods, they were ingesting hundreds of species of bacteria and fungi and thereby subjecting these species to human microbial life processes resulting in a friendly balance or irritation and harm to our tissues. Inflammatory response and immune regulation and identification of these species soon followed. Those that did no harm were left to colonize, and over time established a beneficial relationship with our internal environment. Humans now have a dependency on *Lactobacillus acidophilus* support for the absorption of vitamin B_{12} and as a support in functional digestion of dairy products. *Acidophilus* is the most studied of our friendly bacteria but is by no means the only friendly bacterium needed for digestive balance and function.

There have been a number of recent studies that have found positive correlation between children's consumption of soil and a reduction of the incidence of a number of health concerns, the most important being the development of asthma. These reported studies never link dysbiosis with these benefits, yet I have found in my many years of treating asthma that consistent benefits are achieved by improving the gut ecology. People who have had asthma for a period of time are also inclined to have had numerous antibiotic exposures and cortisone-related therapies as part of the conventional approach to managing this disease.

Friendly microbes include hundreds of species of both bacteria and fungi. Interestingly, in his book *The Bacillus of Long Life*, Douglas only mentioned acidophilus as a normal bacterium of cow manure; all the healthful fermented and cultured beverages from the human cultures the author studied contained non-acidophilus bacteria or yeast. The word *acidophilus* comes from a Greek word meaning "acid-loving." The stomach is an acidic environment, but the small intestine transitions into the basic range and the large intestine is generally neutral. Just as in a forest some species of plants love and thrive in the sun while others prefer shady or wet environments, in your digestive environment there are different microbial populations that do better in each region and in association with dietary habits and microbial food supply. The interrelationship between soil microbes and foods may be a contributor to the benefits seen in the macrobiotic practice and philosophy of nutrition.

Overuse of Antibiotics and Steroids

As a practicing naturopathic physician I have had numerous occasions to prescribe antibiotics and steroids (which promote yeast overgrowth) for the short-term benefit or survival of my patients. I rarely find the need to use antibiotics to reestablish health in my patients. There are times when the amount of life-related stress is so great or when the physical health of the person is so depleted that antibiotics are invaluable. As a whole, I would estimate that I prescribe antibiotics at about 5 percent of the rate of conventional doctors. My therapeutic approach to infection utilizes a number of products and modalities that are much less detrimental than antibiotics. Maintaining a small private practice also allows me to watch and follow my patients' outcomes with an involvement atypical of the high patient volume of modern medicine.

When teaching graduate pharmacognosy in the 1980s, I covered the science of rational antibiotic therapy, which states that preceding the administration of antibiotics there should be the isolation, identification, and determination of sensitivity of the bacterium causing the infection. In this manner the least wide-spectrum antibiotic can be employed, minimizing the destructive effects to the innocent bystanders (the friendly microbes). This philosophy should be the standard used in modern antibiotic therapy, but unfortunately it has become the exception and not the rule. In the rapid-paced practice of modern medicine, it is common to see antibiotics prescribed based upon the system involved and the presumed infectious agents rather than upon the results of culture and sensitivity findings. This practical base of treatment has the benefit of immediate action if the antibiotic is effective against the infectious agent, but frequently results in a much broader destruction of friendly bacteria, creating an opportune setting for the development of secondary problems.

When an infection occurs in a living organism, the site of infection is often inflamed or traumatized so that circulation and delivery of systemic antibiotics is severely impaired. It is necessary to deliver potent concentrations of antibiotics in order to effect complete destruction, or inactivation, of the pathogenic bacterium. The lifesaving properties of antibiotics are absolutely dependent on the delivery of an adequate concentration of it to the site(s) of infection.

New and stronger antibiotics are needed as infectious bacteria develop resistance to the enemies of old. I have found opportunistic fungi that have developed resistance to current antifungals as well. As we continue to up the ante, with stronger and broader-acting antimicrobials, the delicate, nonresistant friendly flora are easy targets of these agents. We are literally clear-cutting our native internal populations, and a host of weeds or opportunistic microbes often take their places. The most common and well known of these opportunists is the fungi *Candida*.

When I used the analogy of a farmer plowing a field and planting a cover crop to prevent the overgrowth of weeds, the corresponding intestinal cover crop for the "plowing" action of antibiotics is a number of friendly bacteria. Unlike the plowing of the farmer, the antibiotics don't plow out the entire crop. Most of the strongest antibiotics have no impact on fungi except for clearing room for additional growth. Similarly, most antifungals have no action on bacteria. This is a logical phenomenon, as it would be inappropriate for fungi to produce protective defense chemicals that harmed their own life processes. Yeasts, like *Candida albicans*, are left intact during antibiotic therapy, with an unchallenged source of food and space to grow. It is like the farmer avoiding all blackberry plants when he plows. When the farmer comes back to plant the crop, the blackberries will not only still be present but they will have spread with each day. The longer we wait after antibiotic therapy to replant friendly bacteria, the more the yeasts will have a stronghold in the gut. As more opportunistic microbes, as opposed to friendly microbes, occupy your intestinal tract, their negative impact on your digestion and health increases.

Some people start experiencing the symptoms of intestinal dysbiosis after only one or two courses of antibiotic therapy. Others are unaware of the low-grade worsening of health and may never find a physician that fully understands their vague, insipid, and individual complaints. Antibiotics that are present in both dairy products and meat also present a much more potent concentration of these chemicals than your friendly bacteria can tolerate. For most Americans, some level of microbial imbalance in the gut is probable.

In the mid-1990s, the CDC (U.S. Centers for Disease Control) issued a warning to American doctors that there exists an alarming overuse of antibiotics in medicine and especially with our children. This resulted in a voluntary reduction of antibiotic prescriptions of more than 30 percent by the year 2000 for children less than sixteen years of age. It is a good start but far from ideal. Prescription of antibiotics should be much lower and more rationally employed. Hopefully this new millennium will bring greater awareness of the harm of antibiotics and a respectful reduction of their overall use.

Environmental Toxins

One other factor that further challenges your intestinal balance is the presence of fungicides and pesticides in your foods, water, and air. It is a certainty that soil-related antifungals cause harm to beneficial gut fungi; it is a probability that they also harm friendly bacteria. Petrochemical-based agents of modern agriculture (fertilizers, pesticides, fungicides, and herbicides) are known to harm important soil organisms involved in creating our topsoils and in delivering soil nutrients to trees and other plants. The EPA puts out regular findings on the pesticide and fungicide content of our commercial foods. Tomatoes and strawberries are typically at the top of the list for fungicides. Cabbage family members always require significant use of pesticides in nonorganic agriculture. It is undeniable that "low" and "acceptable" levels of these chemicals are present in our commercial foods.

The EPA has been active in the investigation of acceptable levels of chemical residue and their influence on human health. In May 2000 the EPA released its initial findings on the most common herbicide used in the cultivation of U.S. corn. It found that the herbicide atrazine, used since 1959, should be classified as a human carcinogen because of its ability to cause breast cancer.[8] The EPA list of chemicals that may contribute to cancer and other serious human diseases continues to expand. Individual associations between single chemicals and human disease continue to emerge, while combination interactions of the hundreds of farm-related chemicals are almost impossible to quantify. Cumulative depression of human detoxification pathways from pesticides and herbicides is only recently being studied and researched. We are far from a complete understanding of the relationships between humans and their consumption of the hundreds or thousands of "safe level" residues within their food. To discuss the benefits of modern agriculture requires a "good faith" avoidance of the many unknowns.

Intestinal Dysbiosis: Diagnosis and Treatment

There are many negative effects of intestinal dysbiosis. There is the obvious loss of cooperative digestion with our friendly flora. There often is an inflammatory process that occurs in the small intestine and results in inadequate protein digestion, the development of food sensitivities, and the production of xenobiotic toxins that can negatively impact your entire body. Each opportunistic organism that sets up residence in your gut can have its own specific impact, and the symptoms and diagnosis of this condition can be quite varied and complicated.

Diagnosis is often a confusing issue. Not only are the opportunists like *Candida* normally present in a healthy digestive tract, though at significantly reduced populations, but the tests of current medicine for stool analysis and culturing are some of the least accurate tests of modern medicine. Often repeated samples are required to finally isolate a single contributory organism, and falsely negative test results are a common occurrence. Fortunately, there are laboratories in the United States that conduct more comprehensive analysis with much greater accuracy of findings. I will occasionally use these comprehensive lab tests, but with their costs often prohibitive, I rely on my own interpretations of a very simple measure of bowel transit time.

Bowel Transit Time

To accurately measure your bowel transit time, simply record the time of consuming one dose of food-grade charcoal and the times that gray or black appears in your stool. Charcoal, when in the activated form, is a highly absorptive molecule that is commonly used to treat bloating or gas. You will find charcoal tablets or capsules at most health food stores as well as at most pharmacies. One or two tablets is the therapeutic dose needed to reduce bloating. Seven to ten tablets are needed to color your stool gray to black. Unlike undigested foods such as corn or seeds that may appear in your stool, charcoal has no irritating action on your intestinal tract, and the color appearance in your stool will most closely approximate your normal transit time. Undigested foods can often speed through as mild irritants and deceive you as to your normal transit time.

There have been many researchers who have tried to establish the ideal transit time for your digestive tract. Realistically, the transit time is associated with the types of foods, amounts of water and fiber, and emotional status (as stress often speeds up the movement). In historical and current study of traditional cultures a transit time of twelve to eighteen hours has often been stated as the ideal. Kellogg wanted to see three bowel movements a day in order to establish an ideal transit. With the highly processed and high-protein diets of modern times, it is unlikely that gray or black color appearing before eighteen hours can be considered normal. I look for a complete transit time of eighteen to thirty hours for those with good dietary habits. Do not be surprised if you see charcoal appearing long after thirty hours even if you have regular daily bowel movements. Often daily habits are eliminating the wastes of meals consumed many days before. The longer undigested foods remain in a 98.6-degree environment, the more decomposition and internal production of irritating by-products occur. Many of these chemicals can and are reabsorbed into your bloodstream, adding to your overall imbalance.

I have done thousands of combination diet-diary–bowel-transit evaluations on my patients. I have predominantly used a tablet form of charcoal marketed by Requa. (Capsule charcoal products usually give very similar results, but depend on the capsule being dissolved for accurate evaluation. If weak digestive processes, such as low acidity in the stomach, don't penetrate the capsule early on, you may not get as accurate information as with a tablet.) By combining a diet diary with the bowel-transit test, types of food and hydration are available for a more accurate determination of the charcoal findings. Proteins need to be broken down in the small intestine for about a six-hour period of time. If your diet is high in protein and low in fluid and water, any show of charcoal before eighteen hours is suspicious. When charcoal appears for multiple bowel movements over more than twenty-four hours, that too is an indicator of imbalance and typically indicates a chronic condition. While not an exact evaluation, the charcoal test has provided me with adequate information for successful treatment of the majority of cases that I have encountered.

Symptoms and Effects of Intestinal Dysbiosis

Optimum health potential can never be achieved with significant dysbiosis. *Candida* and the other opportunists found in dysbiosis can contribute to a whole array of symptoms, and disease conditions may be present on either a chronic or intermittent basis. These can include:

- Arthritis
- Asthma
- Attention deficit disorder
- Chronic fatigue syndrome
- Chronic respiratory infections, post-nasal drip, and excessive mucus production
- Colitis
- Crohn's disease
- Depression
- Dermatitis (rashes), including eczema, psoriasis, and hives
- Diarrhea
- Fibromyalgia
- Headaches
- Inflammatory bowel disease
- Migraines
- Mood swings
- Nausea
- Premenstrual syndrome
- Seizures
- Systemic lupus erythematosis (SLE), or lupus, and other auto-immune conditions
- Urinary frequency

Restoring Balance

Reestablishing normal populations of friendly microbes can be a laborious process, especially if we consider dysbiosis to be a *Candida* condition and neglect to treat the whole environment. *Candida* is undoubtedly a common player in the dysbiosis of antibiotic use, but it is by no means the only organism that creates chronic problems with imbalance. The

"*Candida* diet" and other suggested dietary programs for Candidiasis are often difficult to maintain, provide less nutritional balance and support than is ideal, and finally are flawed in one major consideration: the common exclusion of all food-related yeast during the dietary treatment of *Candida* ignores the immune supportive and nutritional history of beneficial fungi (see Chapter 3.) The exclusion of nutritional and friendly yeast products is somewhat similar to excluding acidophilus during a bacterial infection because it too is a bacterium. Good nutritional balance and habits are important for the complete restoration of health.

To effectively remove unwanted guests from the intestinal tract we need to use a multifaceted approach. The farming analogy provides an excellent overview of the most effective treatment of intestinal dysbiosis. When a field or garden is overgrown with weeds, we need to uproot the weeds, transport them off the field, plant the desired garden, condition the soil, and put up a scarecrow. The human equivalent to this process is as follows:

Weeding We need to use combination products like garlic, undecylenic acid, caprylic acid, *Jugulans nigra*, and many common aromatic herbs. Sometimes it is necessary to include a short course of prescription nystatin if the yeast populations are extensive. When bacterial opportunists are present, berberine (from Oregon grape and goldenseal) is an excellent product of choice. When pathologic bacteria are included in the dysbiosis, the rare use of specific antibiotics may be required. The presence of parasites may also warrant a broader approach, with specific antiparasitic medications, but the vast majority of the people I have successfully treated required no prescription medications.

Removal of Wastes The human wheelbarrow is dietary or supplemental fiber and fluid. Many of the opportunistic microbes of dysbiosis have toxic chemicals within their cells. When we effectively destroy their cell walls, these chemicals are released into the gut. The more supplemental fiber you consume, the more you trap these toxins in the fiber and pass them with normal bowel function. With chronic conditions, which would be revealed by transit times exceeding forty-eight hours, slippery herbs like slippery elm or marshmallow root should be included in the fiber supplementation.

Replanting It is essential to repopulate your intestinal tract with a number of different species of friendly microbes. There are a number of combination products on the market that provide many different species of friendly flora. It is difficult to trust all the manufacturers' claims about the activity of these products because independent evaluation of a product's effectiveness is often absent. Ask the manufacturer about the evaluation process, or talk with your health provider or other authorities to help choose the best available product.

Reconditioning In chronic and acute dysbiosis, the tissues of the alimentary tract are inflamed and often damaged. Essential fats, lecithin, beta-carotene, and a number of normal dietary nutrients are helpful in rebuilding these tissues. Specialized nutritional products are available and often use names that include "leaky gut syndrome" or "intestinal permeability." Rebuilding your intestinal tissues logically follows the completion of the weeding, removal, and replanting phases.

The Scarecrow Secretory function in the gut, which often helps prevent infection, is damaged, reduced, or nearly absent in chronic dysbiosis. Colostrum products serve as some of the best rebuilders of these functions. Licorice root is also an excellent product for improving secretory function.

The length of treatment and choice of treatment elements included is related to each individual imbalance. For single, recent antibiotic use, the process is often only a short weeding and replanting program. For more advanced or chronic conditions the entire protocol is usually needed for at least two months. You will typically experience "die off," or flu-like, symptoms during the height of effective microbial destruction. The weeding, replanting, and removal part of the program should continue at least two weeks after the last symptoms disappear. Symptoms of this phase typically include a short worsening of your individual chronic symptoms.

The ideal diet for this program includes an abundance of whole, organic vegetables, quality sources of proteins and essential fats, and a minimum of caffeine products, processed foods, and simple sugars, including most commercial fruit juices. Canned and processed foods that include rotted or decomposed products (like cheap tomato sauce, juices, and alcohol) can contribute to the inflammatory processes of dysbiosis.

3

Healthy Choices, Personal Empowerment

Benefits Associated with Fasting

People fast for a variety of reasons. Some want to stabilize their eating patterns and know that the reintroduction of foods phase of the fast is ideal for this. Others want to lose weight, improve chronic symptoms, or just feel better. Many people integrate fasting into their general health maintenance plans. Two juice fasts a year, spring and fall, is a recommended maintenance schedule. Still others are combining fasting with other traditional medicines in treating serious health concerns. All of these are valid reasons for considering the fasting diet.

I have been observing the benefits of fasting in both my own experiences and in those of my many patients who have completed the fasting diet. In thirty-plus years of observation I have never seen any serious complications from the fasting process, but I have seen significant improvements in both acute and chronic health problems. It has become my belief that any reversible disease condition can be improved from the enhanced repair processes of a fasting physiology. Many conditions my patients have been told were irreversible have improved from the practice of fasting. Either their doctors mislabeled these conditions or "irreversible" is a term relevant to a certain limited number of therapeutic interventions. This implies that rest, drugs, or surgery do not offer the hope of recovery, only the hope of stabilization.

For many people, the immediate short-term improvements found in their first fasting experience have acted as a springboard to more effective care for their problems. Fasting has empowered them to take a proactive approach to long-accepted maladies. It has reestablished a mental trust in their own innate powers of healing and in the body's ability to communicate the wisdom of a healthy lifestyle.

As discussed in Chapters 1 and 2, there are clear and predictable changes that occur during a fast. Virtually all of these changes result in an improvement of the general health maintenance processes of the body. The ability to remove stored wastes and toxins, the processes of tissue and cell repair, and general immune function are enhanced significantly during a fast. Pain, discomfort, and inflammation are reduced naturally in most fasts. By removing toxic wastes and mediators of inflammation, fasting helps the process of disease reversal. People generally feel better during a juice fast, and they feel better overall after the completion of a successful fast.

Having experienced an improved state of well-being, most people find fasting to be a way to fine-tune their health and improve the natural internal feedback that they have previously ignored. People often come back reporting they have started to feel dull or less vital and know that it's time to repeat a fast. When you know what good health feels like, you are less likely to be satisfied with anything else.

Real-Life Experiences with Fasting

I have seen truly remarkable changes in the health of my patients through the fasting diet and longer fasting programs. Arthritis, dermatitis, arrhythmia, high blood pressure, prostate inflammation, fibrocystic diseases, diabetes, sinusitis, and respiratory infections are but a few of the conditions I have seen improved or reversed through fasting. Some of these stories as well as a few personal stories submitted by past participants are shared in the following pages.

Anecdotal stories serve to personalize the relationship and understanding of fasting in your own health practices. They help to show the successes and fears that people often experience in their personal health care and in fasting. Anecdotes can be misleading, however, and have frequently been used for promotional purposes that don't necessarily represent a balanced view of common experiences. Few of us in the health fields are impressed at the frequent testimonial proof of a new product's "miraculous" successes. We want logic and objective evaluations, not a selective group of testimonials. I provide these stories as unique experiences, but also with the understanding that they are not uncommon testimonials, and are consistent with many shared experiences.

A Case of Fibrocystic Disease

One memorable experience in leading a patient through a fast occurred during my first year of practice. A woman called my office to inquire if I worked with fibrocystic disease of the breasts. She had tried a conventional approach to her condition, which had progressively worsened over the previous five years. She was at a point where she could not lie on her stomach or even wear a bra because of the chronic breast pain. Her fibrocystic condition had advanced so far that her primary physician had referred her for a complete mastectomy. She was reaching out for any options that might prevent this surgery.

She chose to see me after I told her that I had had successes with reversing this condition but it was typically a gradual process. While I told her that I could make no guarantee or promise of success, she chose not to see either of the two doctors who said they could cure the condition in a short time.

We did a thorough history and discussed, in detail, her current lifestyle. I sent her home with a blank diet diary and asked her to honestly record her week's diet, including all food, snacks, beverages, and water. From this initial consultation and the diet diary, it was clear to me that this woman was dealing with a stressful job, and she had very little time for planning or creating a healthy diet. She ate too much fat and too many fried foods, with an excessive amount of coffee and very little fluids. I suggested that she decrease her fat and caffeine intake and try to drink more water as well as add more crunchy vegetables to her diet. I explained the relationships between caffeine, adrenaline, and estrogen and how excessive caffeine and fat intake are promoters of fibrocystic conditions.

After about a month of these changes and taking general supplements, we planned her first fast. She completed a program very similar to the fasting diet and experienced profound improvements in both pain and size of her fibroids. For the first time in many years she was not in a state of chronic pain. Her breasts were much less inflamed and the fibrocystic masses had both shrunk and softened during the fast. While some of the symptoms returned as she reintroduced solid foods, she was by then convinced that surgery was not the only option.

Over the next two years, she fasted a number of times, completely eliminated coffee and created a diet rich in vegetables and with a variety of other quality foods. She also changed jobs and began regular exercise. Over this time her fibroids continued to improve from their original joined mass of about seven centimeters diameter in each breast, to smaller multiple fibroids, then to completely normal tissue. These changes were recorded through mammographic studies and she remains free of masses and free of surgery some eighteen years later.

A Case of Diverticulosis

Another experience involves the case of a patient who came to me through his wife's urging. He was diagnosed with diverticulosis many years earlier and had suffered many acute episodes of diverticulitis (the inflammatory state of diverticulosis) that were treated with steroids and antibiotics. He was in an acute crisis with a colostomy scheduled for the following month. Although he was willing to try a fast, he was by no means convinced that it would help. I modified the pre-fast diet so that he wouldn't have as much fiber and emphasized cabbage, both whole and juiced, which is a traditional medicine for colitis and gastrointestinal problems.

As soon as he entered the juice phase his symptoms began to improve. Pain was reduced, energy was improved, and he felt good enough to extend his fast for a ten-day period. By the end of the juices he was symptom free and tolerated the reintroduction of solid foods with no problems. He began eating a more healthy diet and never had the diseased portion of his colon removed.

Other Conditions Benefited by Juice Fasting

There have been many people in my practice with esophageal reflux, chronic gastritis, irritable bowel syndrome, or colitis who have shown immediate improvements from juice fasting. These conditions and respiratory problems have shown the most rapid and consistent improvements through fasting. Other conditions show improvement, but the digestive tract is obviously the first region of the body to fully experience the restful changes provided by a juice diet.

When a patient presents symptoms of chronic sinusitis, asthma, or allergies, I immediately consider the state of the digestive system. There are no border guards between the mucus tissues of the digestive tract and the respiratory system. Mucus production from an inflamed digestive tract often increases mucus production throughout the body. Typically, as people enter the juice phase, they experience a reduction in mucus production and an opening up of breathing passages. One fasting patient, enjoying the increased sense of smell that comes with most fasts, noticed the sweet fragrance of the spring flowers and then she realized that not only was she not sneezing, but she had forgotten to go in for her weekly allergy shots.

A Case of Heavy-Metal Contamination

Heavy metals are some of the environmental toxins that can be eliminated through the fasting process. One patient of mine, who raced cars as well as owning an automotive shop, came to me, or presented, with a variety of health concerns. For more than ten years he had been in an environment of fumes from solvents, exhausts, and other shop and racing activities. For many years he took little caution in preventing skin contact with these chemicals and did little to improve air quality in his shop and surroundings.

While his environment was filled with fat-soluble fumes and chemicals, it was also a potential source of heavy metals. We performed a hair analysis that revealed a high level of cadmium, which is a harmful heavy metal. Cadmium is added to tobacco, but my patient was not a smoker. The most probable source was in the welding process, which liberates cadmium into the air. We followed the hair analysis with a serum cadmium test to rule out surface cadmium on the hairs that were analyzed. Cadmium was present in high levels in his blood as well.

We chose to do a number of things to attempt to remove the heavy metals from his body. The primary tool was an extended juice fast that was complemented with an herbal decoction (boiled tea) that my patient called "swamp juice," which was made from burdock and dandelion root. He took supplemental zinc, as a competitor with cadmium, and combined niacin and saunas to help excrete the metals and toxins out the skin.

After a two-week fast with nightly saunas, about a quart a day of the "swamp juice," and 100–200 mg of zinc daily, we repeated the serum cadmium test, which reported no detectable cadmium. Hair analysis required the growth of new hair before being repeated. After three months the second hair analysis came back with no detectable cadmium.

My patient has changed welding techniques as well as improving ventilation throughout the workplace.

Fasting provides an improved environment for the elimination of most toxins and wastes. Juice fasting not only provides this improved eliminatory environment but also provides the body with many of the micronutrients needed in the various detoxification pathways.

A Case of Cardiac Arrhythmia

Another patient, with multiple health concerns, presented with a clear cardiac arrhythmia. Her heart would skip a beat on every forth contraction. This arrhythmia would present on an EKG and general exams, making her a logical candidate for a pacemaker. Although we decided to do a fast for other reasons, we noticed that her skipped beat disappeared while on the juices. It returned in a less severe presentation with the reintroduction of foods. A later fast revealed the same improvement and the return immediately upon consumption of potatoes. Most arrhythmias do not respond so dramatically to a short fast. This individualized response was due to an allergic reaction and not due to cardiac disease, showing that allergies can be very deceptive in their symptomatic expressions.

A Case of Rheumatoid Arthritis

A patient of mine persuaded his mother to do the fasting diet as he had successfully completed it on many occasions. Twenty years previously she had been diagnosed with rheumatoid arthritis, and she had been living with pain that was only minimally relieved with her medications. During the fast her arthritis improved significantly and stayed improved until she reintroduced potatoes. Immediately upon eating her first potato, her joints stiffened up and became painful. Without potatoes in her diet she no longer required her pain medicine. Whether she truly had rheumatoid arthritis or whether this diagnosis and the presence of rheumatoid factor and other arthritis-related laboratory and x-ray changes were due entirely to an undiagnosed potato allergy or a combination of the two remains unknown. Without potatoes in her diet her quality of life is significantly improved; for her, this is what truly matters.

Short Juice Fasts and Allergies

The people mentioned above had chronic health complaints that benefited from or were stabilized by short juice fasts. I have seen many people with a wide array of health problems experience recognizable improvements during short fasts. Sometimes the improvements are due to the removal of one or more allergens, but often they are due to other actions of the fast.

Allergic reactions to foods are quite varied. They cover the entire spectrum of the common symptoms of illness. They can produce headaches, mood changes, fatigue, nausea, rashes, shortness of breath, sneezing, diarrhea, achy joints or muscles, and virtually anything you might have experienced when you had a cold or flu. Most of your symptoms of illness are actually sensations of immune function. When white blood cells release immunoglobulins to combat a virus or other microbe, these chemicals have both a specific and a systemwide influence. You may feel achy in every muscle of your body, even though it's a gastrointestinal virus that infected you. It is the same family of chemicals released to fight an undigested food protein that creates the allergic response. It takes many days for the immunoglobulins to be cleared from the bloodstream, so if a food is eaten frequently, there is typically a low-grade expression of these symptoms.

I have included a few comments from patients who have done this fasting program in recent years. Again these are anecdotal experiences, but many of their comments are frequently expressed. The fasting diet is a program that can be done without changing your job or life responsibilities. Roofers, pipe fitters, carpenters, mail carriers, waitresses, school teachers, judges, athletes—the list of occupations of successful fasters in my groups is huge. These people had good energy and great experiences on the fast while handling their normal workload. You can too.

In Their Own Words

Ed

"When I decided to do a fast, I wanted to do it right. I called the medical school, the Chiropractic College, and several doctor's offices, and one name kept coming up—Dr. Steven Bailey. So I made an appointment, and under his care I knew I had done the right thing. When I started on Dr. Bailey's fasting program—called Passage 23—I was surprised to find that one starts out fasting by eating. The first three days you eat a bulking diet.

"It was my decision exactly when to start the fast and for how long. I opted for one week, then at the end of that time, I opted for another week for a total of fourteen days. It was my choice.

"Since I am diabetic I was very concerned about what would become of my blood sugar. By the second day of the fast I had discontinued my glucophage oral medication, my blood sugar was normal, and for the rest of the time it was like I never had diabetes. By the sixth day of eating after the fast was finished, my blood sugar was still normal and my weight loss was still thirteen pounds net. Finally though, I did eventually have to resume my diabetic medicine.

"Altogether it was a delightful experience. Was I hungry? Yes, at times. At other times I forgot I was fasting. I did not change my daily routine. If I went to a social dinner, I just drank fruit juice or water with a slice of lemon. People really didn't care about whether or not I was eating after they got over the idea that I was fasting.

"Sometimes people asked me what I did with all my time since I didn't eat. It was nice to have the free time; usually I tried to go for walks during mealtime. Once in a great while I would get a feeling of weakness so I would just go and lie down. In a short while the feeling would pass and I would go back to my normal routine. I wasn't afraid to lie down if I wanted to. After all, in fasting you have to put your body on nature's operating table, and if occasionally I felt like taking a nap, I didn't care about what anybody else thought. If I were in a hospital I'd be in bed all day, but by fasting I hope to prevent a trip to the hospital by allowing my body to cleanse and heal itself, naturally.

"For those who are so inclined, we remember that fasting is biblical. Many fasts are recorded in the Bible. Also, in the early centuries it was a common method of healing when they didn't have all the modern remedies available now. Animals also fast and rest when they are sick.

"During the fast I felt my mind was clearer. I don't know how to explain it, but it was. My fast was an in-office fast, as opposed to some who do a group fast. I would have liked to have met with a group because there is a benefit in sharing with others, but I just didn't have the time. Dr. Bailey very generously let me do it on my own time schedule.

"To sum up my fasting program I would say I was very pleased and satisfied with this experience in my life. It really wasn't as difficult as I thought it would be.

"I will definitely fast again."

Harold

"Over the years I had done hundreds of fasts and most of them were on water; I had a lot of trouble with them because they were so hard on my body. Dr. Bailey's juice fasts were significantly better and easier on the physical body and made it possible for me to complete the forty-four-day fast.

"Before the fast I weighed 200 pounds and now four years later I weigh 160 pounds and have been able to keep it off. My blood pressure is now normal and my prostate has responded to herbal treatments since I did the forty-four-day juice fast."

Steve

"I'm a forty-two-year-old construction worker. In January of 2000, I went to see Dr. Bailey for a required work physical. Dr. Bailey found that my blood pressure was high, I was borderline diabetic, and I was 100 pounds overweight. I got a real wake-up call. Fortunately, I was with Dr. Bailey.

"In May of 2000 I started juice fasting with the guidance of Dr. Bailey. Though I figured being in construction it would not work for me, I was wrong. In three weeks of juice fasting I lost more than fifteen pounds, gained energy, heartburn ceased, years of long joint aches stopped, and I slept better than I had in years.

"I have watched over the years as some of my coworkers started having the same problems as I did. They saw regular doctors, took medication that had major side effects and was expensive. After taking a bunch of pills they would end up with more problems than they started with.

"I am very impressed with Dr. Bailey's program; in my case, I know it saved me from major health problems and vastly improved my life."

Roy

"I first heard of Dr. Bailey a number of years ago when a friend gave me a copy of his 'nutritional smoothie' recipe. With the successful health results that I experienced on this drink, I decided to attend one of his lectures on health and fasting. I left this lecture being impressed with the way that Dr. Bailey presented himself and especially with the way he unified a great deal of medical information into a usable big picture of health. I have continued to work with him on my own health concerns and have discovered a new level of health in my own life.

"For over twenty years I have been trying to improve my health, with little success. I have seen dozens of doctors who did a lot of laboratory work, but never seemed to get significant results. They would attend to individual symptoms or concerns, with variable results, but never tied the whole picture together. Dr. Bailey has continued to work with me as a partner in health and with amazing success. He has helped me to build and evolve my understanding of health practices with an integration of traditional and contemporary medicine.

"I have found that Dr. Bailey embodies the principles that he presents. He has treated me with compassion and respect and has served as a pillar of strength when needed. I spent over ten years working at the Oregon Health Sciences University and have noticed these same qualities in the best researchers and physicians that I have been around. He clearly comes from the heart and actively seeks to educate and empower his patients. Instead of trying to get more and more patients or to sell a product, Dr. Bailey works to get his patients healthy enough to free themselves from regular medical needs. His passion for natural medicine, his humility, and his caring for people have provided me much support in my own journey to health.

"I have been guided though a number of fasts by Dr. Bailey. My first fast was in the spring of 1996. In the first week of his juice fast, called Passage 23, I felt better than before I started. By the second week of juices, I had more energy than since I had been a teenager. By the third week I didn't know if I wanted to eat solid foods again, as I felt so good. My skin had cleared, I was more flexible, and my achy joints were nearly free of pain. The improvements from my first fast lasted for about one and one-half years with better energy, clearer eyes, improved sense of taste and smell, improved breath, and a better fat/muscle ratio. Most importantly, I felt more connected to my body and had a clearer understanding of how the body, mind, and spirit work together.

"I now call his group fasts my 'Spring Celebration' of renewal and rebirth. As I have always enjoyed a good celebration, I've never been able to go less than five weeks on his juice programs. I, myself, know of hundreds of people who have gone through his one-week program with beneficial outcomes and no serious problems. I have only had positive experiences with my extended fasts and have always been able to do better with my day-to-day work needs than while eating my normal diet. While on his fasts I have unloaded shipping crates in 100-degree weather, chopped and moved multiple cords of firewood, cleared acreage of fall debris, and worked full time in a physically demanding field.

"Each time I've done a fast, my experiences have been different. Dr. Bailey has provided me with alternate juice programs (the 'Master Cleanser') and has led me through complete water fasts. He has occasionally provided me with massage, physiotherapy, and spinal manipulations to assist my healing process. While you may not have the benefits of being a personal patient of Dr. Bailey, you now have the basic framework of his fasting programs. So, it's time to celebrate, get cozy, relax (as the technical and safety issues are well addressed), and begin your journey from disease to 'ease.' Life is a great ride and this is the guidebook to 'ease' you along your way."

Diseases and Other Conditions That Can Improve with Fasting

My personal experience, my readings, and the experience of my patients lead me to believe that nearly every chronic and acute health problem can benefit from juice fasting. Unlike water fasting that has many contraindications and special considerations, juice fasting has very few restrictions. If it is a voluntary and informed desire to fast, only pregnancy and breast-feeding are conditions that I would exclude from the fasting diet. Diabetes is a condition where competent self-management or supervision is required. Most other conditions are dependent only upon the physical capabilities of following the program.

The conditions I have seen improve with fasting are an A–Z list of most diseases. These improvements are a result of a number of physiological improvements that occur during a fast. While these have been outlined in Chapter 2, they deserve mention in relation to disease reversal.

- Fresh vegetable juices contain more vitamins, minerals, and enzymes than the normal diet.
- Fresh vegetable juices are virtually self-digesting. This leaves additional energy in the form of oxygen, general blood flow, and

the nutrients and calories used by the normal digestive processes. This energy is now available for other repair and maintenance processes.

- Food sensitivities and allergens are removed.
- Fat and salt are reduced in the bloodstream, leading to improved circulation.
- Removal of stored toxins is enhanced.
- Immune function is enhanced as well as normalized.
- Mood and energy are often improved.

These processes work together with a rejuvenating effect. Inflammation is reduced, immune function is fine-tuned, and cell repair is enhanced. If the body has the ability to improve or reverse a disease condition, its actions are typically enhanced by juice fasting. The improvements are measurable both clinically and subjectively. You will recognize the improvements, and that is typically all the science that one needs to further one's interest in and practice of fasting.

While most health conditions show benefits from juice fasting, there has been a historical appreciation of particular vegetables or fruits for particular conditions. There is also the ability to use herbal, fungal, or homeopathic products without disrupting the fast. These can be used according to their indications, provided they are neither high-protein nor druglike in their actions.

Juice Choices by Conditions

When a long list of fruits and vegetables follows a condition, it is not necessary to combine them all in the same juice. Carrot mixes with celery, beet, and cucumber as a good base to combine with most other vegetables. You generally don't want to combine fruits with vegetables, although Dr. Norman Walker was famous for his carrot-apple combinations. As you may have noted, the same vegetables come up for most health concerns. Carrot, celery, and beet, which are the foundation of the fasting diet, are listed for nearly every health problem. Add a little cucumber, spinach, and garlic and you've covered most of the recommended juices for all of these common problems.

Use a juicing machine to extract the juices from fresh vegetables. Carrot juice can be drunk straight, but as a general rule celery and cucumber should make up 50 percent of a combination, beet juice should not exceed 33 percent, and other vegetables and herbs should be used to taste at no more than two to four ounces per quart. Fruit juices, when diluted 50 percent with water, can be used in any tasty combination.

Consume the juices immediately, or you can refrigerate them for up to forty-eight hours.

Acne Apricot, asparagus, beet, carrot, cucumber, grape, green pepper, lettuce, raw potato, spinach, yellow dock

Allergies Beet, carrot, celery, cucumber, raw potato

Anemia Beet, carrot, celery, coconut, dandelion, fennel, horseradish, lettuce, nettle, parsley, pomegranate, spinach, turnip, watercress

Angina Beet, carrot, celery, hawthorn, parsley, spinach

Arthritis Beet, carrot, celery, cucumber, grapefruit, nettle, spinach

Asthma Carrot, celery, garlic, grapefruit, horseradish, lemon, parsley, potato, radish, spinach, watercress

Biliousness Beet, carrot, celery, cucumber, dandelion, nettle, parsley, spinach, watercress

Bladder disease Carrot, celery, cranberry, cucumber, parsley, spinach

Boils Beet, carrot, celery, cucumber, garlic, lettuce, parsley, spinach, yellow dock

Bronchitis Beet, cabbage, carrot, celery, cucumber, dandelion, garlic, horseradish, lemon, pineapple, radish, spinach

Cancer Apple, broccoli, cabbage, carrot, celery, fungal extracts, garlic, spinach

Colds Beet, carrot, celery, cucumber, garlic, grapefruit, horseradish, lemon, orange, radish, spinach

Colitis Apple, beet, cabbage, carrot, cucumber, papaya, spinach

Conjunctivitis Carrot, celery, endive, parsley, spinach

Constipation Apple, beet, carrot, celery, cherries, cucumber, potato, prunes, spinach

Cystitis Beet, carrot, celery, coconut, cranberries, cucumber, green peppers, parsley, spinach

Dermatitis Apple, beet, carrot, celery, cucumber, parsley, watercress, yellow dock

Diabetes Brussels sprouts, carrot, celery, endive, green beans, Jerusalem artichokes, parsley, spinach

Diarrhea Apple, beet, blackberries, cabbage, carrot, celery, garlic, nettle, papaya, parsley, pineapple, raspberries, spinach

Eczema Beet, carrot, celery, cucumber, parsley, spinach

Esophageal reflux Cabbage, carrot, celery, marshmallow root, slippery elm

Epilepsy Beet, carrot, celery, cucumber, parsley, spinach

Fatigue Apple, beet, carrot, cucumber, lemon, lettuce, orange

Gastritis Beet, cabbage, carrot, cucumber, lettuce, papaya, pineapple, spinach

Gout Beet, black cherries, carrot, celery, cucumber, parsley, prunes, spinach

Headache Apple, beet, carrot, celery, cucumber, lettuce, parsley, spinach

Heart disease Carrot, celery, cucumber, garlic, hawthorn, parsley, spinach

Hemorrhoids Carrot, spinach, turnip, watercress

Hepatitis Beet, black radish, burdock, carrot, celery, dandelion root, garlic

High blood pressure Beet, carrot, cucumber, garlic, parsley, spinach

Impotence Apple, beet, carrot, celery, cucumber, lettuce, parsley, spinach

Influenza Beet, carrot, celery, garlic, horseradish, lemon, radish, spinach

Insomnia Beet, carrot, celery, cucumber, grapefruit, lettuce, spinach

Kidney problems Beet, carrot, celery, coconut, cucumber, dandelion greens, grape, lemon, parsley, spinach, watercress

Low blood pressure Beet, carrot, celery, cucumber, parsley, spinach, watercress

Migraine Beet, carrot, celery, cucumber, dandelion, parsley, spinach

Nervous disorders Beet, carrot, celery, cucumber, lettuce, parsley, spinach

Obesity Beet, cabbage, carrot, celery, cucumber, spinach

Prostatitis Asparagus, beet, carrot, cucumber, lettuce, spinach

Psoriasis Beet, carrot, celery, cucumber, parsley, spinach

Renal stones Beet, carrot, celery, cucumber, parsley

Sciatica Beet, carrot, celery, cucumber, parsley, spinach

Sinusitis Beet, carrot, cucumber, garlic, horseradish, lemon, onion, papaya, pineapple, radish, spinach

Tonsillitis Apple, beet, carrot, celery, cucumber, lemon, orange, parsley, pineapple

Toxemia Beet, carrot, cayenne, celery, cucumber, garlic, parsley, spinach

Tumors Beet, carrot, celery, cucumber, spinach, turnip, watercress

Ulcers Aloe, beet, cabbage, carrot, cucumber, spinach

Varicose veins Beet, carrot, celery, cucumber, grapefruit, parsley, spinach, turnip, watercress

Supplements

Fresh, organic vegetable juices are exceptionally nutritious. There is generally no need for most people to supplement a juice fast with vitamins, minerals, or other natural products. Vitamins and minerals are concentrated as solid vegetables are transformed through juicing into a tasty, biologically active drink. Most of the indigestible fiber is removed in the juicing process, reducing the original mass or bulk to about one-third while releasing the natural plant enzymes stored within the fibrous structures. These enzymes give fresh vegetable juices a short refrigerated "shelf-life" of little more than forty-eight hours with reduced nutritional content even at this time. Just as these enzymes aid in the digestion and absorption of juices, they increase the natural oxidative breakdown of many of the nutrients found in the juices themselves.

The use of supplements during a fast should be thought out from a variety of considerations. Is it a choice of necessity or an option, in what form is the supplement, and what are its intended as well as complete actions? Necessity speaks to why you are doing the fast. Are there some safe supplements that might add benefit to your specific health needs? The form or composition of the supplement is a consideration that looks at whether there will be additional digestive and absorption requirements. For example, many vitamins are protein- or fat-based molecules that stimulate pancreatic and gastric functioning at levels not required in the juice diet.

Concentrated proteins and fats change the chemical and physical environment of a fast. During a fast, there is a resting environment that takes place throughout the digestive system. The body acclimates to its available energy sources and maintains a balance throughout normal activities. Reawakening with abrupt increases in digestive and metabolic activity can significantly alter this normal fasting environment. High levels of protein intake during a liquid fast can lower post-fast metabolism, stimulating weight gain instead of normalization. Proteins and fats also activate hypothalamic and other glandular responses that alter energy and metabolic systems throughout the body. Vegetable juices have quality proteins at a level that doesn't demand significant digestive response, especially as they are accompanied by the plants' own proteolytic enzymes. As a rule, supplemental foods that are high in protein or fat should be used sparingly during a fast.

Herbs

Many herbs can be considered as foods and juiced into your cocktail blend with your vegetables. Garlic is an excellent example. It is used as a food in many common dishes but is also taken for its liver and immune support as well as its cardiovascular and antifungal actions. Black radishes, burdock, and dandelion roots are also long-revered herbs or foods for liver support. Their actions are primarily those of a food, antioxidant, and anti-inflammatory, whereas dandelion greens have a potent diuretic effect and must be respected for their strong pharmacological actions. Herbs like peppermint, ginger, and cinnamon are also common culinary herbs that stimulate the release of digestive juices in the mouth and stomach. These herbs can aid digestion, while not altering the fasting environment.

There are also herbs that have a true drug influence on the human physiology. *Guarana*, a common energy and weight loss herb, is 5 percent caffeine, higher than coffee. Ephedra, called "Mormon Tea" in American history and "Ma Huang" in Chinese tradition, is also a potent stimulant and is much more druglike than foodlike in action. Some herbal products are even stronger acting than caffeine or ephedra or, worse, may be toxic with even small doses. The FDA maintains a G.R.A.S. (generally recognized as safe) list that includes herbs with primarily subtle or foodlike actions. When in doubt about an herb's actions or relative safety, either seek an authoritative review or avoid the unknown risks. As a rule, herbs should be in a liquid form or powdered form mixed with liquid. You do not want to take tablets or capsules during a juice fast.

I have used herbal tinctures with many people on the fasting diet. Herbs like *Echinacea, Grindellia,* and licorice can be helpful for sinusitis and respiratory problems. I've used *Echinacea,* saw palmetto, and diuretics like uva ursa with chronic prostatitis. Powdered larix has worked well for glandular swellings. Most of these conditions will improve during a successful fast without additional support. When in doubt about the appropriateness of a product, just follow the basic guidelines and enjoy the natural benefits.

Fungi

Mushrooms and fungi have a long history of nutritional and medical use. They do not juice well raw, yet they have easily absorbed nutrients when delivered as liquid or powdered extracts. As a whole food, mushrooms typically provide quality proteins, fiber, and carbohydrates. Mushrooms like shitake have been shown to improve human cardiovascular function, hypertension, and cholesterol levels when consumed regularly as part of a normal diet. The area of greatest current interest and research is the fiber-bound polysaccharides.

Polysaccharides are large carbohydrate molecules, like the starches in potatoes and rice. They are typically broken down into simple sugars and used for energy. It takes time for the starch-digesting enzymes of your mouth and pancreas to free up the simple sugars, which makes polysaccharides and starches an ideal "steady energy" source. Some large polysaccharides, like those found in *Coriolus versicolor, Lentinula edodes, Ganoderma lucidum,* and *Grifola frondosa,* are known to be absorbed intact into the human bloodstream. These intact polysaccharides have exhibited a wide range of beneficial properties.

In the early 1990s I was introduced to an Oregon mycologist who proceeded to tell me about an amazing mushroom extract from Asia that had proven benefits for cancer and a number of other human diseases. He told me that this extract of the fungus *Coriolus versicolor* was extensively researched, written up in hundreds of journals, and widely used in the treatment of cancer in Japan and other nations. I was exceptionally skeptical that there existed a product of this much effectiveness and study that was virtually unheard of in North America. The product was called PSK or Krestin, and journal articles about this drug were abundantly available.

As I researched *Coriolus* I found that there were more than four hundred journal articles with nearly one hundred presentations of human controlled studies in the medical literature. Journals like the *New England Journal of Medicine* and *The Lancet* had published studies about PSK that reported significant benefits in the treatment of cancer and in reducing the side effects of chemotherapy. The fate and distribution, toxicity and safety, and standards of assay for potency and action were all well documented. Although safe, effective, and complementary to standard American medicine, this important natural drug was not available to the American public.

My skepticism was replaced with respect for *Coriolus* and a number of fungal extracts. I joined with the mycologist and a research chemist who specialized in biochemical assay and helped form JHS Natural Products. JHS began importing *Coriolus* extracts in the mid-1990s and has expanded to include a number of varieties and forms of fungal extracts. Working with this company I have continued to study and increase my knowledge of medicinal fungi. I have traveled to Japan and China; met with patent holders, researchers, and doctors who have used these products; and visited manufacturing facilities in both Japan and China. As my knowledge has grown, so too has my admiration and respect for the much-underutilized benefits of the fungal kingdom.

The primary class of chemicals that represent these well-researched fungal medicines is a group of polysaccharides called beta-glucans.

These very large and heavy-molecular-weight polysaccharides have been shown to increase human immune function through a variety of pathways. Receptor sites for beta-glucans have been identified on human macrophages, although the immune benefits extend into killer-cell activity, T-lymphocyte number and activity, and thymus and spleen neogenesis in animal-based research. These immune benefits translate into improved cure rates and times of remission in a number of human cancers as well as improvements in hepatitis B and chronic hepatitis.

While I have found these polysaccharides to be well tolerated and beneficial during fasts, they must be made available to humans through hot-water extraction. Fungi, as a distinct class of life, have cell walls that are comprised of the rigid structure chitin. This substance is the same fiber that makes up the shells of crabs, lobsters, and other arthropods. The polysaccharides are primarily attached to the chitin cell walls, and your digestive enzymes do not release them in the raw form. It takes temperatures in the 80–100 degrees Celsius range to break the chitin attachment and release the polysaccharides for human availability. This is why mushrooms don't juice well and why, since many commercial products are not heat extracted, there is great variability of fungal products on the American market.

The predominant body of contemporary human research on the benefits of medicinal fungi involves concentrated hot water extracts of these products. The dose of these extracts often is very close to the dose achieved in traditional Asian medicine through hot-water infusions (teas) taken frequently. There are standards of manufacturing, extraction, and constituent assays that can lead you to an informed use and dosage of these products. Just as in herbal preparations and vitamins, it is your right to ask a manufacturer about assays for potency, contamination, and general or specific approaches to quality control.

There are many beneficial actions that have been identified from both edible and medicinal fungi. These benefits encompass a wide array of common diseases including cancer, hepatitis, AIDS, diabetes, hypertension, and heart disease. It is logical to assume that our western avoidance of mushrooms in the standard diet helps to increase our rates of illness; it is evident that the inclusion of a variety of mushroom extracts in your diet helps to reverse many of these same diseases. From a preventative standpoint it would therefore be wise to include a wide variety of mushrooms in a normal diet so that we don't have to treat the results of their absence at a later time.

Keep It Simple

The carrot, celery, and beet combinations recommended in the fasting diet are powerful aids to an effective fast. It is typically not necessary to add herbal or supplemental products to a juice fast to observe benefits. I recommend that you keep your first fast simple and not get too creative. Herbal teas like peppermint, hibiscus, and chamomile are considered normal fluids, and additional vegetables like cucumber, spinach, burdock root, or garlic are also freely included.

4

The Awakened Spirit

---

*"Science without religion is lame;
religion without science is blind."*

—ALBERT EINSTEIN

Aligning the Body, Mind, and Spirit

As I wrote in Chapter 1, I believe that the only separation that exists between the body, mind, and spirit is of an entirely arbitrary nature. Only through the limited logic of the conscious mind and ego are we able to create a duality between body and spirit. We have begun to isolate the physical chemicals associated with emotions, feelings, and mental processes. We have, once again, begun to understand that how we think impacts how we feel and how we live.

Fasting is, without question, both a spiritual and a physical process. For those people who have successfully fasted in the past, this unity is self-evident. For the first-time faster, this relationship will present itself clearly in the form of a quiet, yet fully awakened spirit. Fasting and prayer are used interchangeably throughout the Bible, and while there are true water fasts described in this text, many times the term "fast" reflects the discipline of mental focus consistent with deep prayer as well as true fasting.

By engaging in intentional fasting, you are aligning your body, mind, and spirit. You can aid this process by thoughtful creation of the ideal environment during the fast. Finding time to walk in the woods, visit the river, the ocean, or other natural places is one way to help your fasting environment. Avoidance of television and other forms of media is often encouraged by practitioners of fasting. Not only will you avoid the current trauma of our world, you will also avoid the constant advertising for fast foods, quick-fix pharmaceuticals for unhealthy lifestyles, and the constant prodding for unnecessary material purchases.

Most people do not have the opportunity to attend a retreat or spa for their fasting experience. My fasting program is a "working class" fast that should allow you to keep up your normal work and exercise programs while still enjoying the benefits of a fast. There will still be job stresses, traffic congestion, and other negative experiences, but hopefully you can help minimize the detractors of your physical and spiritual balance.

The Science of Inner Healing

We are just beginning to integrate the power of the mind into the Western paradigm of medicine. Psycho-neuro-immunology is a term that emerged in the late '80s as a result of research into the subtle influences that can be observed between immune function and one's state of mind. Without doubt, emotions such as fear and anxiety have been linked to diminished health and understandable negative changes of digestive, cardiovascular, and immune health.

The field of biofeedback, which refined its techniques in the late '60s, was one of the first "modern" Western medical acceptances of the power of mental awareness, or the mind, to influence health. These techniques were used primarily to influence the adrenal response to stress through awareness, and thus provide positive feedback to the imbalanced state. It remains a useful tool in the management of pain and the control of certain stress-related conditions.

We are far from understanding the complete relationship between the spirit, the mind, and the nearly unlimited power of the body to heal itself. Contemporary authors like Deepak Chopra, M.D., have written on the receptor sensitivity of all cells to the chemicals of emotions. There is a long journey ahead before we are able to more completely study and map out these relationships, but the old writings of disease-personality associations are proving much more relevant than recent skeptics have maintained. The future science of medicine will undoubtedly place a greater emphasis on how we think, what we think, and how we can support or replace the current tools of healing through meditation, prayer, and mental discipline.

Visualizations, Affirmations, Meditation, and Prayer

Visualizations, affirmations, meditation, and prayer are first cousins of the same family. Any or all of these techniques or practices can be employed to aid in your personal well-being. For using them to revamp your life, there are some important guidelines to be aware of.

One of the most important things to consider is the widely understood principle that the spirit and the subconscious minds were not created within the confines of the English language (or other contemporary dialect). The spirit is experiential and symbolic. The power of the word, in its limited interpretation, can often derail the most carefully chosen objectives.

Here is an exercise that I use when lecturing or when discussing this concept with patients. I ask people to close their eyes and not to think about a polar bear. Not to think about the white snow and white bear. Almost always people are smiling or laughing as they open their eyes, just having seen a mental picture of a polar bear as their eyes were closed and their ears open. Negative words, within spoken language, have no symbolic meaning. Your mind and subconscious immediately seek out the symbol and imprint that picture in your mind. You can imagine the confused state that exists within, when you pray or affirm that you do not want cancer, heart disease, or any other condition that you fear or wish to avoid. It is important to accentuate the positive.

When you desire an improved state of health you should implant healthful images or concepts. Instead of thinking about the many bad things that you wish to avoid, focus on the states of health that are desired. Instead of affirming that you do not want cancer, state that you want a long, healthy, vital life. Choose the positive image or concept that most aligns your healing powers.

Another problem that many people face is found in their own self-images. When people are living with guilt or a sense of worthlessness, it is hard to accentuate or even accept the concept of the grace of healing. I have found the following exercise to be a useful springboard to a more forgiving attitude.

I ask people to imagine that they are walking on a sunny, beautiful woodland trail. I ask them to imagine that they see a deer standing in the distance. What do you feel or experience is my first question. Typically, people respond positively, that they see beauty and are thankful for this special moment. Never once has someone said that the deer had a bad hair day, that if the deer just lost ten pounds, it would look better. Never once has someone questioned whether the deer was a good spouse, a good role model for its offspring, or whether it had lived up to its potential. It is so easy to see beauty in nature, yet see only critical reflections in your own mirror. If only we each could see our own miraculous truths.

I have often said that if songbirds had human brains, only one in ten would be willing to sing in public.

These are two of the most important concepts in effective practice of visualization, affirmations, meditation, and prayer: to understand the power of the word, and to accept that you have a right to accept and seek out your basic needs. There are many different approaches to these spiritual practices. Certainly it is possible to use these tools in a self-centered, ego-based manner, especially as the difference between needs and wants remains confused in many minds. Many forms of meditation emphasize that you should clear your mind of all thoughts, and many faiths state that prayer should seek God's will and not seek human desires.

The power of the word or mental intention is an elusive study. We, as well as science, cannot separate this power from our study of human health and disease. When you choose to take a proactive approach to your health, like jogging; choosing your foods more wisely; engaging in meditation, practicing yoga, or other practices, you are aligning your mental processes with the vision of improved health. Your confidence in a particular practice or approach is directly related to the clarity of mental intention. Even the classic "double-blind study" of Western medicine creates a doubt in the minds of those participants who know they might be receiving a placebo. And the power of the placebo is to a large degree a minor reflection of the power of the mind and spirit.

To take the double-blind study into a more scientific approach, participants would, by intention, be unaware that they are in a study, and would be confidently given their medicines or placebos by experimenters who also were unaware that there was an experiment taking place. Fasting, by definition, could never be subjected to a true double-blind experiment. Likewise, nearly all of our current scientific research ignores the truly remarkable power of the spirit and mind to influence health.

There are a great many books, tapes, and videos that can assist you in developing a comfortable relationship with the techniques of meditation, affirmations, visualizations, breathing, and prayer. No one technique is right for everyone, so trust your inner wisdom about what feels right for you, and therefore will work best for your true needs.

Environment is an important part of successful practice. Most people need to find a safe, quiet, and comfortable setting to maintain focus in these practices. I encourage you to be thoughtful of your environment, yet, as described in Thich Nhat Hanh's *A Guide to Walking Meditation*, every step you take, and every breath you take, can be meditation if you maintain a wakeful consciousness.

Breath is also an important component of successful meditation, and it can aid in the other practices as well. Expanding your breath to a full, deep natural rhythm not only helps calm the mind and body, but also has many positive influences. I was very impressed with a recent book on the subject of breathing called *The Tao of Natural Breathing*, by Dennis Lewis. The breath can be a powerful friend or foe, depending on how you practice. Certain breathing techniques, even those with a long history, may complicate your practices if you are far removed from the natural breath.

One of my favorite everyday techniques of breathing meditation was introduced to me by Irving Oyle, M.D. He presented it as the "I am" breath, and to date it has proven itself as one of the easiest, positive techniques I've encountered. It can be done with eyes open, and in nearly any setting. Taking a full, deep breath, you think or say, "I am," followed as you exhale with the quality you wish to empower. Words like calm, happy, energetic, healthy, and peaceful are examples of qualities you might choose to encourage. The next time someone passes you on the right, only to make you brake as he or she takes the next left turn, try breathing "I am calm" instead of reacting to the person's rudeness. Do you really want the rude or insensitive actions of others to manifest as your own unpleasant state of being?

Only you will know what practices serve you best. Do your best to integrate practices that honor your values, provide beneficial results, and can be maintained for the long term.

The Seven Chakras

Part of my naturopathic practice over the years has included the physical medicines of massage, physiotherapy, and spinal manipulation. In examining spinal positions, muscle tensions, and holding patterns of my many patients, I have come to appreciate how the physical symptoms of distress consistently mirror the emotional and spiritual difficulties of the individual I'm working with. The relationships have very simply expressed themselves within the emotional and spiritual attributes associated with what are known as the *chakras* of the affected regions of the body. Often these relationships have prompted me to delve more deeply into the emotional and life issues that often remain unspoken. It is not uncommon for a spinal misalignment that has been resistant to standard manipulation or adjustments to easily release after the patient has integrated awareness of these relationships into his or her conscious thought.

Over the years I have studied many different systems of life energy, from the Western sciences of biology, chemistry, physics, and special relativity to traditional medical models, cultural and religious systems, as well as more esoteric models. The energy of life is an acknowledged mystery in nearly all systems of medicine and religion. Our Western roots look at biologic forces and the early Greek acknowledgment of a vital energy, a life force. The Chinese speak of *chi* and *Qi*, the Indians speak of *prana*—others of God's, the Creator's, or the Goddess's energies—and all acknowledge the incomplete ability of the conscious mind to totally comprehend or measure these forces.

There are many systems that attempt to incorporate these energies into the functional diagnosis and treatment of disease in humans. The meridian energy of acupuncture, the vital force of homeopathy, the universal consciousness of Jungian psychology, the energy of foot reflexology, Kirilian photography and Russian medicine, the Science of Mind of religious metaphysical practice, applied kinesiology of Western physical medicine, and the chakra energies of Ayurvedic and native medicine are some of the better known fields that I've studied. Of all the systems, the chakra system has served me best. It is consistent with the Gaia theory (earth as a living organism) of current times and has enhanced my understanding and treatment of patients.

Those who believe in this system of life energy generally recognize seven major chakras. There are many minor chakras said to be associated with life energy, but I find simplicity and a functional applicability dealing with the major seven. These major seven areas of energy have been represented with similar locations, colors, and functions throughout many different traditional cultures. They have been found in historical drawings and sculptures in Asian artifacts as well as island and American tribal art. This cross-cultural similarity may speak to the truth of these energy fields or may speak to early mysteries shared by our ancestors. For whatever reason, this system has fit remarkably well into my private practice over the years.

Just as in Chinese medicine, the chakra system is based on the belief that the life energy flows throughout the body, feeding and being fed by other energy currents. In acupuncture a primary goal is to balance these energies and allow unrestricted passage from one meridian point or channel to another. Similarly, when one chakra is closed to receiving energy from or allowing energy to flow to another region, a state of energetic and hence physical, mental, emotional, and spiritual imbalance exists. Balancing the energy flow leads to a much more vital life experience, and to what we term vibrant health.

Human Relationships Within Chakras

The colors, emotions, and importance of each chakra region of the body are represented in Figure 4.1, a comparison diagram of the chakras. This is of course a rather simplified discussion, but it may provide you with enough of a foundation to review your own tensions, back pains, or other physical distress in a manner that offers a new approach to your own health needs. There are many different interpretations or meanings of the various chakras. I provide my thoughts and the meanings that have proven most useful to my practice.

The chakras are located in the center of the body, ascending from the first or root chakra, located in the pelvis, to the seventh chakra, which actually is positioned over the top of the skull. They are attributed colors in the spectrum of the rainbow, which begin in the reds at the first chakra and end in the violet or purple of the sixth. The seventh chakra, or spiritual gate, is the white light or halo-like glow portrayed in our representations of angels. When you are in balance, you are thought to be emitting a rainbow of spiritual light.

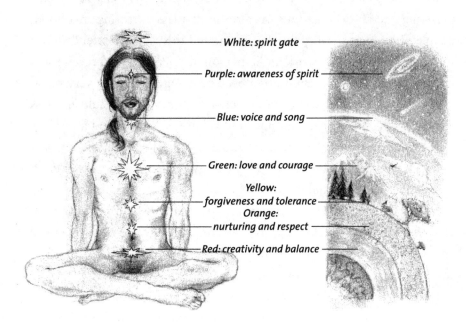

FIGURE 4.1 *The Seven Chakras*

The first chakra, with the color red, represents both life balance and creative energy. In the emotional and spiritual interpretations, balance simply refers to whether you are setting your own priorities, and whether your day-to-day activities and labors honor these priorities. Creativity is both the physical act of procreation as well as the creative artistry of human endeavor. If your occupation is a painter or musician or other creative pursuit, these job-related efforts might not satisfy the creative needs of your spirit. Detaching your creative outlet from purposeful intent is needed to refuel this energy.

The second chakra, the color orange, is located between the umbilicus (belly button) and the spine and represents nurturing, trust, and respect. Often this important life experience, found in the unconditional love of parents for their children, is absent or limited in your actual childhood experiences. When you are not adequately nurtured, you may find this energy imbalance presenting itself in many ways. Obvious associations would include fear of abandonment or isolation as well as problems digesting and absorbing foods. As a result of a less nurturing childhood, people often become very self-sufficient, and this is often extended into life as a task-oriented, workaholic personality. People who receive less unconditional love as a child often become caregivers, being very sensitive to the pain and needs of others. Self-sufficiency often results in a less receptive environment for support and acknowledgment and also leads to relationship choices of partners who are in need of care.

As I mentioned above, the healthy energy of one chakra fuels or energizes the adjoining chakras, both above and below. In the case of a depleted second chakra, this may result in impaired support of the third chakra, which can lead to a hypercritical or judgmental nature. The third chakra, the color yellow, lies in the deep region of the solar plexus (where the ribs come together above the stomach). The healthy energy of this region represents the qualities of forgiveness and tolerance. Imbalance reflects the shadowy qualities of judgment and criticism. Like the Chinese liver meridian condition of an "overheated, rising, arrogant liver," anger and judgment are not only shared with others, but reside within your own being. This can lead to excessive self-judgment, which in turn limits your ability to accept love (fourth chakra) and to accept nurturing from others (second chakra). When treating heated or inflamed conditions of the liver, like hepatitis, discussing the patient's qualities of forgiveness or tolerance with him or her can be important in helping the patient to move out of the chronic state.

The fourth chakra, the color green and often called the "heart chakra," lies in the region of the heart and represents the qualities of love and courage. Imbalance or insufficiency results in the inability to receive love, in fear, and in sadness. Anxiousness, fear, sadness, a sinking heaviness, depression, or even chest pains may lead you to consider your ability to accept love from others and yourself. Love is a true need of healthy people, and it begins with self-love. Trust is needed to be open to love, but a so-called act of love that expects some return to the giver, even when implied versus stated, is not love, but a social exchange with costs. Love and virtue are their own rewards. As you learn to respect and forgive your human limitations, you are less vulnerable to the hidden costs of manipulative affection.

The fifth chakra, the color blue and called the throat chakra, represents the ability to speak and to be listened to. It lies directly between the mind and the heart, representing the convergence of what Scott Peck, in *The Road Less Traveled*, calls the longest journey in the human experience. To unify your mental and spiritual energies with the heart energy, as a song or voice, is indeed a common human challenge. The heart is afraid of hurting someone with words while the mind is unwilling to remain silent.

The sixth chakra, the color purple, is considered your awareness of your spirit and your oneness with all life. It is located between and behind your eyes, and, as the pineal gland, was called the "seed of the soul" by the famous scientist and doctor Paracelsus. As you accept your oneness with life and spirit, you can gracefully accept and provide for your needs with an understanding that humans need creativity, balance, nurturing, forgiveness, love, and freedom of expression as much as plants or animals need air, water, sunshine, and food. When you understand your true emotional and spiritual needs, you are on your way to a much healthier and more fulfilling life.

The seventh chakra, the white light of life, is considered a gateway from the heavens. If you accept your spiritual identity in your sixth chakra, you are open to receive this white light energy from the heavens.

As you probably have noted, the colors red, orange, yellow, green, blue, and purple are the visible colors of the rainbow. When you are in balance, you are thought to be emitting a rainbow of light. The colors of the rainbow spectrum are the same as the color changes going from the center of earth to the heavens. The Gaia theory looks at the earth as a living organism and has been expanded by some to be the belief that all life shares or is a hologram of this planetary organization. While the U.S. EPA has stated, "The planet is a living system, and we need to protect it,"[1] the Gaia theory has been embraced by people such as Deepak Chopra and Stephen Hawking as they merge relativity with life sciences.

The core of the earth is, of course, theorized to be molten red. The infrared energy of our planet's core is measurable and is considered to feed into the meridians of the feet in the Chinese system. It is logical to think that this earth energy also feeds into the first chakra. The crust around the core represents the color orange, speaks to the metaphor of nurturing, as in the womb, and has led some people to suggest that this area, instead of the first chakra, represents creativity. The soils of the earth are in the yellow spectrum, providing a base for the green world of plants, which with their oxygen feed the energy of the heart and lungs. Just as the plants reach for the blue sky, our visible sky is the color blue with the outer atmosphere transitioning into the purples. The sun, moon's reflected light, and stars represent the white light of the heavens and like the red core energy of our planet is recognized in acupuncture as a source of energy for the yin meridians of the hands.

Henry David Thoreau wrote that it was important to walk barefoot on the soil and to sleep on the ground, not elevated on a bed. Many traditions have emphasized the benefits of walking barefoot, and if only for better foot health, this might be a valuable practice. Your breath clearly feeds the lungs and green heart energy, and your openness to spirit allows you to receive the white energy from above. You can disregard this discussion if it doesn't feel right. It is certainly not a necessary belief or practice for the purposes of experiencing a successful fast.

The qualities that I have mentioned are, I believe, needs of our species. You need balance, creative outlets, nurturing and respect, forgiveness and tolerance, the ability to give and receive love, the freedom to express yourself, and finally that knowledge that you share spiritually with all life and creative forces, as you know them. If you accept or expect that your needs will not be met, you will not live to your physical, emotional, or spiritual potentials.

Journaling

In my fasting guidebook, *Passage 23*, that I have given to my fasting participants, I have left ample room for notes and journaling. This is especially important for recording the post-fast allergy testing, but it has great value both during the fast and throughout life. Recording your daily experiences and feelings is itself a form of meditation, calling upon a wakeful consciousness of your day-to-day life. As you record and observe your own relationships between actions, thoughts, feelings, and end results, you are empowering yourself with the knowledge of positive change. Often as you look more clearly at your own thoughts and actions, you are freeing yourself of the need for therapists, doctors, and other expensive practitioners of the healing arts.

5

Fasts for All Reasons

Juice and Water Fasts: A Comparison

The human history of fasting has been comprised primarily of water fasts. As a spiritual practice, as a rite of passage, and as a therapeutic tool, fasting in our traditional experience means water only. There is no question that water-only fasts are the most powerful of all fasting practices. It is my respect for this power that makes me such a proponent of juice fasting in modern times. For the person reared in a Western environment, the water fast with its accelerated release of toxins may prove too strenuous or even harmful. While I advocate water-only fasts, I feel that you should work your way to water fasting with juice fasts, improved dietary habits, and detoxification supports.

There are many programs devised for both juice and water fasting. There are also many different "semi-fasts" using fiber supplements, raw foods, protein powders, and modified intake of solid foods. Some of the modified fasts may actually promote changes associated with starvation, leading to post-fast weight gain and a worsened level of health. The beneficial changes of fasting can be most easily accomplished through juice- or water-only programs. From a health maintenance and general safety viewpoint, I advocate vegetable juices, the "Master Cleanser" (discussed on page 89), or water fasting as the best choices.

The primary objective of a fast is to provide the body with as few digestive requirements as possible, while stabilizing energy through supplemental and alternative energy sources. These alternative energy pathways include the conversion of stored fat into usable fuel and the recycling of cellular nutrients through the process of autolysis. Autolysis simply means "self-digestion." It is the highly efficient, combined processes of the white blood cells, liver, spleen, and kidneys as we "digest" our old and dead tissues, recycling in the bloodstream those intact components of cells such as minerals, fats, and vitamins for reuse, while eliminating unusable cell wastes. This process is aided by the fasting physiology. As long as increased fat conversion and accelerated autolysis are occurring, the detoxification and rejuvenation of fasting is present. Elimination of released toxins is a necessary component of all fasting programs and is supported by adequate intake of fluids and water. In comparing fasts, this volume is quite varied; appropriate volumes are discussed when a particular protocol is outlined.

I have outlined the fasting diet in Chapter 6 with inclusion of preferred juices. While carrot, celery, and beet are common vegetables used in a variety of juice-fasting programs, they are by no means the only beneficial juices and some of the other choices are mentioned in Chapter 3. The fasting diet uses two quarts vegetable and one quart fruit juice on a daily basis. This combination allows the benefits of fresh organic vegetable juice (alkalinity, excellent nutrition, and detoxification support) while still allowing a change of cuisine. Many people tire of vegetable juices when they are the only beverages consumed. It is not necessary to include fruit juice in this program, but the one-quart volume does not lead to an acid environment like with a fruit-juice only fast.

Fruit juices, when consumed in undiluted form, can create blood sugar swings similar to eating refined sugar. This fact leads to the obvious solution of diluting your fruit juices with water at about a fifty/fifty blend. This diluted combination will allow for a more normal delivery of sugar and avoid the hyperglycemic/hypoglycemic swings of straight juice.

It is estimated that the sugar of apple juice will be absorbed eight times as quickly into the bloodstream as will the sugars of an apple consumed in its whole form. While an apple a day may keep the doctor away, the juice of an apple is not nearly as beneficial.

Fresh-squeezed fruit juices contain a number of helpful nutrients including vitamin C, bioflavinoids, and a wide array of natural antioxidants. Once a juice has been canned or pasteurized, these nutrients are nearly all depleted through oxidative breakdown. When you are consuming fresh vegetable juices, the antioxidants and vitamins of the fruit juice are minimal players in the overall nutritional program. While it is better to consume fresh, unpasteurized fruit juices, their part in the fasting diet is primarily as fuel and a change of taste. Bottled fruit juices are acceptable for this program.

In general, fruit juice fasts are less beneficial and more difficult than either vegetable juice or water-only fasts. The acid-producing quality of fruit juices is counterproductive to the many acidic detoxification pathways of the body. This can lead to less effective elimination of wastes and more overall discomfort during the fast.

Fruit juice fasts are more appropriate when done in warmer weather as they will tend to cool the body. This is true of all fasts, but even more important in fruit-juice-only fasts. The chemically based digestive processes associated with a normal diet produce significant heat. This thermal by-product of digestion contributes to your warm-blooded core body temperature. When you fast you have to replace this free heat with internal heat production, which requires caloric support. In cold temperatures the normal energy demands of heat maintenance can compromise the energy balance of the fast.

The Master Cleanser

One fruit-based fasting program is both gentle and effective. This program is popularly called the "Master Cleanser" program and uses lemon juice combined with cayenne pepper, maple syrup, and water. This fast is gentle as compared to a water-only fast in that the maple syrup provides easily absorbed fuel allowing a slower conversion of stored fat into fuel and thus limiting the release of toxins to a manageable level. The healing crisis that may accompany a water fast is not typically seen in this program so that most people can continue normal activities as they do this program.

The Master Cleanser does not require the inclusion of enemas as is necessary for vegetable juice fasts. It is also a better "mucus reducer" than vegetable juice fasts. The concept of mucus-producing foods is common to a number of different traditional forms of medicine including the Ayurvedic medicine of India. In Western medicine, Dr. Arnold Ehret developed an entire system of cure based on his "mucusless diet" and fasting. He lectured and wrote in the early 1900s about the mucus cause of disease in humans and stated in his book *Rational Fasting*, 1910, that "Civilization has brought a greater cleanliness on the outside of the body, but an awful uncleanliness inside."[1]

Dr. Ehret recommended that people follow a mucusless diet for up to two years before attempting a water fast and also recommended that most people can benefit from drinking a combination of lemon juice and honey during a fast. This is an early form of the Master Cleanser; the cayenne pepper and maple syrup were added at a later time. This program is often added or included as part of longer fasts by my patients. Here is the recipe for the Master Cleanser.

Master Cleanser Recipe

The juice of 2 organic lemons
⅛–¼ teaspoon cayenne pepper (organic preferred)
2 tablespoons pure maple syrup (organic preferred)
Filtered or distilled water (enough to make 1 quart total liquid)

Mix lemon juice, cayenne pepper, and maple syrup. Dilute mixture with the filtered or distilled water to one quart. (Some recipes dilute to one pint.)

You are asked to consume six quarts (or pints) of this combination per day. For the quart mixtures, this is all you have to drink each day. For the pint combinations, it is recommended that you consume an additional two to three quarts of water per day. If you are in the juice phase of the fasting diet, you may choose to switch directly to this combination to give yourself a break from the vegetable juices, to extend the program, or just to experience this fast. If you are planning to do this fast as a single program, the pre-fast diet of Chapter 6 can also be used before entering the Master Cleanser protocol.

Water Fasts

Experience and knowledge or competent supervision is a requirement for water fasts. They are more stressful than either vegetable juice fasts or the Master Cleanser. There are many spas and healing resorts that specialize in water-fasting programs. The experience of these clinicians is critical in understanding and supporting the healing crisis that may occur while fasting on water. Your overall state of health and degree of toxicity are related to how severe or stressful a water fast can be. Just because you feel okay doesn't mean that you can breeze through a water fast without supervision.

There are a great many facilities around the world that specialize in water-fasting programs. Just as in juice-fasting programs, there are many variations to these regimens. Pre-fast diets vary as do the amount and type of fluids consumed. Some programs allow vegetable broth for electrolyte balance; others monitor electrolytes and supplement minerals or broth as indicated. Otto Buchinger's programs (now continued by his daughter) in Spain and Germany allow one cup of coffee in the morning for those individuals with low energy and blood pressures. I know of one fasting program published by an English naturopath that allows a glass of table wine in the evening for his fasters. As a rule most water-fasting programs do not allow coffee, alcohol, juices, or other supplemental fluids or products. The human body "knows" the water fast and needs little support to achieve the detoxification and rejuvenating benefits of the fast.

Physiologic Changes and Benefits of Fasting

Water fasts have been the most studied and scientifically explored form of fasting. The science of fasting is most easily quantified through a water-only program as all nutrient-related variables are eliminated. The physiologic changes and benefits that occur during a water-only fast have been observed for thousands of years. In more modern times we have been able to measure chemical, microscopic, and cellular change information that was not possible in earlier centuries. These changes are predictable and to a large extent are also present during juice fasts.

One of the first changes that occurs during a fast is the body's use or consumption of glycogen stores from the liver and muscles. As outlined in Chapter 6, if you do a pre-fast diet like the one described, the glycogen reserves are utilized prior to the onset of true fasting. If you go from a normal diet to a water-only fast, you will see this process occur in the first twenty-four to forty-eight hours of the fast. These are the times that hunger is most present. When the body is tapping into its reserve energy, it has not yet appreciated the intention of the fast and your appetite centers seek to reinforce eating. This increased appetite naturally decreases by day two or three.

With the reduction of glycogen reserves comes a natural decrease in serum glucose, which results in a decreased production of insulin from the pancreas and the beginning of stored fat liberation and conversion throughout the body. This fat liberation and conversion reaches its maximum on the third day, which is typically the hardest and least comfortable day of fasting. Proteolysis, the breakdown and conversion of protein into fuel, becomes an added energy support for the brain and body. This proteolysis primarily occurs from connective tissues, serum, and diseased growths or tumors. This energy cycle is significantly reduced in the juice fast, as are the increased eliminatory processes required by this process.

Electrolytes are generally conserved during a fast. It is important to drink adequate amounts of fluids to allow the body to regulate electrolytes adequately. Occasionally people will have a lowering of potassium or calcium in a prolonged fast. These important minerals can easily be monitored during the fast and replenished with clear vegetable broth or other mineral support.

Laboratory values vary considerably between individuals on the same fast. Typically serum glucose is reduced and blood clotting is reduced, as are many inflammatory indices. Many lab values reflect the individual's changes and don't follow an exact pattern. Serum cholesterol and triglycerides are often elevated during a fast due to the fat conversion that is taking place on an accelerated basis. These values and others will commonly move to a healthy normal status after the fast. Extended vegetable juice fasts typically show a reduction in serum cholesterol and triglycerides during the fast phase as well as post-fast.

Natural wastes, such as ammonia, from this increased energy activity will be elevated in the urine. Toxins from the environment will also reveal themselves in the urine and feces. It is very important to drink enough water to allow these wastes and toxins to be eliminated in the most dilute form possible.

Water fasts have been shown to improve a number of common health concerns and diseases. Arthritis patients show consistent improvements with water fasts as short as six days.[2] Some of this may be due to food allergy associations with arthritis or to digestive inflammation and its association with arthritis, but there are many controlled studies that have shown consistent and sustained improvements to all aspects of arthritic symptoms.

Most people think about weight loss as a primary benefit of fasting, and this is indeed a common occurrence. Americans are an obese group of people with many problems associated with diet, lifestyle, and weight.

I think of good nutrition and exercise as the most important factors related to obesity, and generally try to work with diet before and after fasts even when they are specifically done for weight-loss purposes. Fasting can and has often been done for weight-reduction purposes. If you lose weight through a fast and return to a highly processed and refined diet, your weight probably will return.

Throughout the past hundred years studies have been conducted and reported on therapeutic fasting. Conditions that have shown benefit from fasting include diabetes, mental disease, allergies, skin diseases, cardiovascular disease, gastrointestinal diseases, liver disease, chemical poisoning, and the already mentioned arthritis and obesity conditions.[3] Fasting, whether water or juice, provides an environment wherein the body can perform its repair and maintenance processes in the most efficient manner. The list of diseases that can benefit from fasting is almost every condition known to medicine.

Juice fasting is much less severe than water fasting. Juices provide supportive energy while significantly reducing digestive function. They provide nutrients that aid the liver and kidneys in detoxification processes and allow you to perform normal activities. This is not true of the water-only fast. Most people need to significantly decrease their physical, mental, and emotional energy to do well on a water fast. The Buchinger Clinics do not allow television, news, or other media exposure that might agitate or interfere with the resting state of the water fast. Even on juice fasts it is nice to reduce stimulation from outside sources like the television and media to allow focus on the events within the body.

Fasting from Historical and Cultural Perspectives

The Buddha fasted, Christ fasted, Mohamed fasted; whether your religious roots are in Buddhist, Christian, Muslim, Hindu, Jewish, or Native

American philosophies, your tradition includes a clear appreciation for and avocation of fasting for both therapeutic and spiritual purposes. Fasting is a highly revered practice of discipline and therapy in traditional Western and Eastern medicines. It is believed to predate written history as part of the spoken word, tribal mysteries, and knowledge of early societies. Finally, it is an innate natural wisdom of the human body.

While society and our external environment have changed immensely in the past one hundred years, our bodies have changed very little. The need for fasting is perhaps greater now than ever before. Conventional medicine and science seek a silver bullet to solve the diseases caused by our lifestyles, dietary imbalances, and accumulated dangers of job and environmental exposures, while telling us to keep doing what we do. We are advised to quit smoking, exercise, eat a low-fat, low-salt diet, practice safe sex, get our immunizations, and have regular physical exams. These guidelines are not attempting to eliminate the known causes of cancer, heart disease, and other Western diseases, but to monitor and treat their inevitable occurrence.

Millions (perhaps billions over time) of humans have fasted on juices or water with abundant observation of its many benefits. It is not a radical, unsafe, or unfounded therapy or practice. It is an exceptional experience that benefits the body, mind, and spirit. Your HMO or private doctor is unlikely to direct you toward fasting. They are unlikely to challenge the average American diet and inadequate nutritional recommendations of conventional medicine. It is up to you to take an affirmative and proactive approach to health.

Most people that I have taken through fasts have fasted again, often on a regular basis. Most patients making positive changes in their diet, nutrition, and lifestyle have noticed significant improvement in energy, resistance to acute illness, and overall well-being. These changes have led to increased personal awareness and generally a better long-term diet and lifestyle. I encourage you to keep an open and objective mind when you try the fasting diet. You should be able to perceive if you have more energy, feel better, and are doing better in general after the fast. Your own experience will help you understand the long religious and cultural traditions of fasting.

Contemporary Fasting Programs: Their Benefits and Contraindications

As we become more aware of the many dangers of our toxic environment, a great increase in detoxification products in the health and medical industries has followed. Obesity, a major American health concern, has seeded the growth of the weight-loss industry. Many of the weight-loss programs and products are both safe and beneficial, while many products utilize stimulants and an unhealthy long-term approach to health. It is hard as a consumer to make an informed choice, particularly when there are so many different promised solutions for your own concerns.

I have tried to outline some of the basic principles of fasting and detoxification throughout this book. Hopefully these principles will help you to evaluate the various products and fasting programs that you encounter. Evaluate as best you can, and listen to your body's response if you try a particular program. You have rights and responsibilities that should be your companion throughout all your health choices; use these to your own benefit in appraising facilities, fasting programs, and products.

One of the most important principles of medicine is "do no harm." The most important consideration in evaluating a particular program is understanding the potential risks. For detoxification products, this risk appraisal involves review of the ingredients, the manufacturer's evaluation of purity and consistency of ingredients, and your individual relationship with these products. Have there been any human studies conducted with a particular product? For facilities, the appraisal might include who is the director, what are his or her credentials and experience, how long has the program been conducted, and what are the outcomes of the participants?

The human body does most of the work of detoxification and rejuvenation during a fast. It is not necessary to get elaborate and complicated in your approach to fasting and detoxification. Simple and basic fasting programs can achieve remarkable results and are the best starting place for the inexperienced faster. As experience grows or need dictates, advanced approaches to fasting can be safely integrated.

6

Dr. Bailey's
Five-Day Power Fast

I began leading groups on extended juice fasts in 1983. The program I used with my associate Elaine Bayes Gillaspie, N.D., was very similar to the one I employ today and that is outlined in this chapter. We used to call this program a working-class fast as it did not require the cessation of normal work or exercise programs. It is a program that generally provides enhanced energy while still invoking the beneficial changes of the fasting physiology.

There are three basic phases to most fasting programs. These are a pre-fast diet, a fasting phase (water, juice, etc.), and a staged reintroduction of foods. You will find considerable variations in how different practitioners design these phases and also will find agreement from most that there are conditions and situations where immediate entrance into the fasting phase is indicated. For most intentional fasts a pre-fast diet is recommended to prepare the body, liver, and especially the intestinal tract for minimal to no daily fiber, as well as for the enhanced elimination of toxins experienced with most fasts.

The program outlined in the following pages accomplishes the important needs of the pre-fast diet, discusses the appropriate juices and elimination supports of the fasting phase, and parallels a smooth transition into healthful nutrition with simple yet informative food allergy testing. Unlike water-only fasts or other more severe programs that require competent guidance for most people, this vegetable and fruit juice program has proven easily achievable for thousands of people. Hopefully you can use it and the information of this book to begin or expand upon your own use of fasting for health maintenance and for therapeutic purposes.

While the entire program is outlined in this chapter, I would strongly encourage you to read the entire book before embarking on this fast. There are many things throughout this book that will help you create the optimum experience and to understand and embrace the process with more confidence and enthusiasm.

Basic Guidelines

Probably the single most important principle of fasting is that it must be voluntary. This not only means an active intention on the part of the participant, but also the knowledge necessary to safely and effectively engage in the fast. Knowing when to cease a fast and how to deal with individual problems encountered during a fast are critical to the ease of a successful fast. Just as fasting is one of the most basic forms of natural healing, nature has its ways of communicating its wisdom to the individual faster.

Another guiding principle of most fasting programs is not to share or tell people that you are fasting. This is sometimes impractical and obviously not relevant to fasts of a symbolic or public nature such as hunger strikes or protest fasts. The traditional reasoning behind this guideline is that fasting has been a spiritual discipline and most practices advocate prayer and fasting as a private and certainly not a boastful act. In our current times a second reason for not telling people you are fasting is that many people will translate the word *fast* into starvation or deprivation and will unnecessarily encumber your experience with fear and often confrontational judgments. If and when family or friends do share their concerns and opinions, remember that behind their comments is often a genuine concern and caring for your welfare.

Until you have successfully completed a number of fasts it is generally good to follow the specific guidelines of the intended fast as closely as possible. Creating your own special features for a fast may prove beneficial, but should only be done when they are consistent with the natural principles and philosophy behind fasting. I have tried to be very specific in outlining the general instructions and requirements of each phase of the power fast. I have also mentioned options and adjuncts that can be utilized within the framework of this program. Whether it's the fasting diet or any other program, the most important advice is to listen to your own body and its communication to you about your practice. Your own health and welfare always takes priority over rules and intentions.

Fasting is always both a physical and a spiritual practice, regardless of one's spoken purpose. Even when you are planning a fast for spiritual reasons, it is important to honor the physical laws of the body and of the changes that occur during a fast. For this reason fasting should be done with the intent to provide the most ideal physical, emotional, and spiritual environments possible.

Some of the important things to consider are the quality of your food, water, and juices; the social and home settings that you surround yourself with; and your general lifestyle choices during the fast. The quality of food and juice are discussed in greater detail in the nutrition chapter (Chapter 7), but the simple rule is "fresh and organic" as much as possible. Water should be of a high quality, either filtered or distilled. Take time to review and consider your social and family calendars so that you don't find yourself in mid-fast with an important wedding, get-together, or other activity that will compromise your program. Try to incorporate both a healthy lifestyle and supportive activities such as exercise, yoga, meditation, prayer, massage, hydrotherapy, affirmations, and visualizations. Finally, take pride in and keep a good attitude about the positive changes that you are engendering.

There are times and situations where a fast is not appropriate or should be ended earlier than intended. Contraindications for fasting vary by type of fast and by author. For the fasting diet the only absolute contraindications are excessive fear of or apprehension about fasting; pregnancy; and lactation. I have successfully supervised people on fasts with virtually every major disease condition. For insulin-dependent diabetes and advanced, severe disease states, I would recommend supervision whenever possible but I know the power fast to have been very beneficial to many people with these conditions.

The Pre-Fast or Bulking Diet

This pre-fast diet is designed for the fasting diet, but I have found it to be a useful practice for a number of fasting protocols including the Master Cleanser and water fasts. There are a number of objectives to the pre-fast diet and they include the following.

- Cleaning the intestinal tract with high fiber—primarily raw foods and supplemental fiber
- Eliminating most fat and protein from the intestines
- Reducing glycogen stores in the liver
- Optimizing liver and gall bladder status
- Eliminating unhealthy choices and practices

The standard pre-fast diet is three days in length but can be extended when appropriate. Reasons for extending may include excessive coffee intake that requires a longer cessation schedule or a low-fiber standard diet that makes the high-fiber qualities of the recommended diet too severe or uncomfortable. The vast majority of people that I have supervised in fasting have done quite well with this three-day, high-fiber program, but listen to your body and use a little common sense. If you eat a large amount of processed foods, meat, and dairy and a small amount of crunchy vegetables, fresh fruits, and whole grains, you may wish to reduce the volume of food and fiber and extend the number of days on the pre-fast diet. Likewise if you get uncomfortably bloated or experience cramping or nausea with the first day of the program, reduce and lengthen as well.

Each of the three bulking days begins with a traditional liver/gall bladder tonic called the liver flush. This is a drink comprised of three tablespoons good quality olive oil, one to two cloves of garlic, and the juice of one lemon, and optionally recommended, the juice of one orange. The garlic should be diced or minced, and the entire drink can be stirred or blended (blending gives it a more oily, salad-dressing taste); the desired actions of this tonic are similar in both forms.

Olive oil, like most pure oils, acts as a chologogue, a term meaning "increases the flow of bile." When your body receives this drink with its high fat content into the empty stomach, the chemical, neural, and glandular response is to anticipate that even more fat is on the way. This neurochemical response stimulates the gall bladder to contract and the liver to produce additional new bile to aid in the digestion and absorption of the expected fat. By fooling the body into thinking you just ate a whole moose, the liver and gall bladder respond more dramatically than for normal meals. This increased response accomplishes a number of desired changes in preparation for the fast.

When bile is released into the intestinal tract for normal digestion, it encounters and mixes with the digested fats within the food. Acting similarly to soap in its ability to mix fats in water, bile is reabsorbed in the distal third of the small intestine where it helps carry fat in the saline bloodstream. Between 90 and 95 percent of bile is reabsorbed and eventually stored in its conjugated form in the gall bladder.

The higher the dietary fiber, the lower the reabsorption percentage. Since bile is comprised of water, salts, and then cholesterol, fatty acids, and lecithin, here lies the primary theorized action of the relationship of dietary fiber to lowered cholesterol. The more fiber in the diet, the more cholesterol is eliminated with the digestive wastes. In the bulking diet the liver tonic is followed in one-half hour with vegetable fiber, water, and a bowel tablet, and then a half hour later with a high-fiber, low-fat fruit breakfast.

With this protocol a much higher percentage of the bile is eliminated, and even though the liver is responding each morning with the production of new (unconjugated) bile, there is also a daily reduction in the volume of stored bile. This feature might prove important in long fasts and particularly in the protein-powder weight-loss "fasts" of conventional medicine, which have reported a high incidence of gall bladder problems with extended programs. In addition to reducing stored bile reserves, traditional medicine theorizes that the significant elevation of bile flow within the liver results in decongesting the tissues of the liver. This in turn increases normal blood flow, oxygenation, and hence, general liver activity. For the purposes of therapeutic fasting, the better the liver functions, the greater the ease and benefit of the fast. I have found this drink to be well tolerated by my patients and only occasionally accompanied by nausea or other symptoms. If you have had your gall bladder removed, have difficulty with fatty foods, or have other known liver problems, you should reduce the olive oil to two tablespoons.

As I mentioned above, the liver tonic is followed by one teaspoon of vegetable fiber (psyllium husk powder is recommended), one bowel tablet (ask for a gentle laxative product at your health food store), and eight to sixteen ounces of water. This fiber, laxative, and water routine is repeated pre-lunch and pre-dinner.

Breakfast is an all-fruit meal while lunch and dinner are to be all vegetable. A daily program is listed below with ideas on variety and quantity. One vegetable meal can be steamed, especially in colder weather, but raw is preferred.

THE PRE-FAST DIET

Upon Rising

The first thing taken each of the three bulking days is the liver tonic mentioned above. It should be consumed as directed prior to water, tea, or any other foods or fluids. In this manner the action of the olive oil on the liver and gall bladder is enhanced.

Mix or blend the following ingredients:

- 3 tablespoons of good quality olive oil (1½ if you have cronic liver problems or if your gall bladder has been removed)
- 1 to 2 cloves of fresh organic garlic, diced or pressed
- Juice of 1 lemon
- Juice of 1 orange (optional but recommended)

The liver tonic is followed in one-half hour with the first of three daily fiber supplements. I have used psyllium husk powder for this purpose for my clinic program since its inception, but you may use equal amounts of your own favored product if you have one. Psyllium powder is used in a large number of commercial fiber products and is more concentrated than ground psyllium.

Daily Fiber Supplement

- 1 teaspoon psyllium powder
- 2 to 4 ounces juice or water
- 1 gentle herbal laxative
- 1 to 2 8-ounce glasses water

Mix psyllium powder in juice or water and drink. Follow this with the laxative and glass(es) of water.

Breakfast

A fruit breakfast is to follow at least one-half hour after taking the fiber and laxative. This allows the fiber to pass through the intestinal tract with the bile and olive oil, rather than with the breakfast fruits.

You are free to substitute equivalent amounts of any fruit for the examples mentioned below. Choose the freshest, highest-quality fruits but also choose those that are most appealing to you.

- 3 unsulphured prunes
- 1 peach
- 1 banana
- 1 to 2 apples
- Herbal tea, water, or diluted fruit juice as desired

Snacks

Because the bulking diet is very high fiber and low calorie, you may still find yourself with an appetite in spite of the large amount of food you are consuming. You are free to snack on whole fruit, raw vegetables, raw sunflower seeds, or diluted juices between your scheduled meals.

Pre-Lunch

At least one half hour before lunch, you are to repeat the fiber, laxative, and water supplement mentioned above.

Lunch

Lunch and dinner are both vegetable meals. One may be steamed or both can be completely raw. They may be identical meals or as varied within the vegetable kingdom as you choose.

Clean and prepare in large salad bowl:

- ¼ bunch green lettuce (not iceberg)
- ¼ bunch spinach

- 1 medium carrot
- 1 celery stick
- 1 medium tomato
- ¼ to ½ cucumber
- ½ cup sprouts—any kind
- 1 to 2 green onions
- 1 to 2 tablespoons raw sunflower seeds

Add nondairy salad dressing of choice, primarily using oil, vinegar, lemon juice, garlic, and herbs of choice. You can substitute any like quantity of vegetable for any of the above salad ingredients.

Pre-Dinner

At least one half hour before dinner, repeat the fiber, laxative, and water supplementation mentioned above.

Dinner

Dinner may be an identical repeat of the lunch salad, or you may choose more variety, maybe even some vegetables you've never tried before! Some options to consider include endive, watercress, mustard and other greens, parsley, radishes, jicama, and peppers, as well as mushrooms like shitake, morels, or portobello. Cabbage family members like cabbage, cauliflower, broccoli, kale, and Brussels sprouts should be steamed rather than raw for this phase of the program.

Fluid Intake for the Pre-Fast

I recommend that you consume at least three quarts of fluid per day during the bulking phase. This amount includes the one to two eight-ounce glasses of water that you take with the fiber supplement, so if you drink two glasses of water each of the three times you take the fiber, you have one and one-half quarts of fluid left to consume throughout the day. For the purpose of the pre-fast diet, you can count water, mineral water, herbal teas, and diluted juices toward this goal.

This is by far the hardest and most cumbersome part of the entire fast. For my groups I always arrange for the first day of bulking to be on a Saturday so that most people will be initiating this routine on a nonwork day. Each day gets a little easier as the routine becomes familiar. It is still a lot of food and very few calories or energy. This is an intentional component of this program so that you deplete your stored sugar reserves and therefore enter the juice phase with fewer food cravings and a faster initiation of the fasting physiology.

If you can't eat all the recommended food, just do your best. You don't need 100 percent compliance to proceed into a successful fast.

The Juice Diet

The power fast uses a combination of fresh vegetable and fruit juices. On the normal program each person consumes two quarts of vegetable and one quart of fruit juice daily. Additional water, herbal tea, or juice is taken daily to achieve five to six quarts of total fluid. I have included the nutritional information for the basic vegetable juices that I recommend, but choice of juices for specific conditions comes from traditional indications and use versus a contemporary association of micronutrients and disease states.

For the power fast I suggest a fifty/fifty or two-thirds to one-third blend of carrot and celery for one quart and a second quart that is one-third carrot, one-third celery, and one-third beet. The choice of fruit juice is mostly for a change of taste and additional calories. Juices should not include citrus or tomato and should not have additional sugar or chemicals added.

An important point: beet juice will be expelled from the body as a bright red color that looks very similar to fresh blood. It will also often color your urine pink. Do not fear that you have uncovered a bleeding condition in the colon or a urinary tract infection. This color is due to the colored pigments in the beet, and the presence of this color in urine or feces is a normal occurrence.

The following tables represent the nutritional values in juices.

TABLE 6.1 RECIPE ONE—CARROT, CELERY

	½ CARROT	½ CELERY	TOTAL
Calories	216.1	91.2	307.3
Protein	5.0	4.1	9.1
Fat	2.1	0.4	2.5
Carbohydrates	44.3	17.8	62.1
Calcium	169.0	178.2	347.2
Phosphorus	164.5	127.9	292.4
Magnesium	105.1	100.5	205.6
Iron	3.1	59.4	62.5
Sodium	214.7	575.8	790.5
Potassium	1558.3	1558.3	3116.6
Beta-carotene	50270.0	1096.8	51366.8
Vitamin B$_1$	0.2	0.1	0.3
Vitamin B$_2$	479.8	0.1	479.9
Vitamin B$_3$	2.7	1.3	4.0
Vitamin C	36.5	41.1	77.6

TABLE 6.2   RECIPE TWO—CARROT, CELERY

	²/₃ CARROT	¹/₃ CELERY	TOTAL
Calories	264.2	60.0	324.4
Protein	6.6	2.7	9.3
Fat	2.8	0.2	3.0
Carbohydrates	58.9	11.9	70.8
Calcium	224.7	119.3	344.0
Phosphorus	218.7	85.6	304.3
Magnesium	139.7	67.3	207.0
Iron	4.1	39.7	43.8
Sodium	285.5	385.7	671.2
Potassium	2072.5	1044.0	3116.5
Beta-carotene	66859.1	734.8	67593.9
Thiamin	0.2	0.0	0.2
Riboflavin	638.1	0.0	638.1
Niacin	3.5	0.8	4.3
Vitamin C	48.5	27.5	76.0

TABLE 6.3   RECIPE THREE—CARROT, CELERY, BEET COMBO

	¹/₃ CARROT	¹/₃ CELERY	¹/₃ BEET	TOTAL
Calories	144.2	60.2	140.7	345.1
Protein	3.3	2.7	4.8	10.8
Fat	1.4	0.2	0.3	1.9
Carbohydrates	29.6	11.9	29.7	71.2
Calcium	113.2	119.3	48.0	280.5
Phosphorus	110.2	85.6	99.0	294.8
Magnesium	70.4	67.3	75.0	212.7
Iron	2.0	39.7	2.1	43.8

	⅓ Carrot	⅓ Celery	⅓ Beet	Total
Sodium	143.8	385.7	180.0	709.5
Potassium	1044.0	1044.0	1005.0	3093.0
Beta-carotene	33680.9	734.8	60.0	34475.7
Vitamin B₁	0.1	0.0	309.0	309.1
Vitamin B₂	321.4	0.0	0.1	321.5
Vitamin B₃	1.8	0.8	1.2	3.8
Vitamin C	24.4	27.5	30.0	81.9

Table 6.4 Recipe Four—Cucumber, Cabbage, Garlic Combo

	½ Cucumber	½ Cabbage	Garlic (3 cloves)	Total
Calories	41.0	67.6	12.0	120.6
Protein	2.0	5.5	0.6	7.56
Fat	0.2	0.4	trace	0.6
Carbohydrates	7.8	10.5	2.7	21.0
Calcium	57.5	154.1	3.0	214.6
Phosphorus	62.1	124.2	18.0	204.3
Magnesium	25.3	0.0	0.0	25.3
Iron	2.5	2.0	trace	4.5
Sodium	13.8	50.6	3.0	67.4
Potassium	368.0	618.7	48.0	1034.7
Beta-carotene	575.0	460.0	trace	1035.0
Thiamin	236.9	0.1	101.0	338.0
Riboflavin	0.0	0.1	trace	0.1
Niacin	4.6	0.6	trace	5.2
Vitamin C	25.3	126.5	trace	151.8

Why Vegetable Juices?

I have found vegetable juices to be the ideal nutrition for both the new and experienced faster. By drinking fresh vegetable juices, you are getting high-quality nutrition with minimal digestive effort. The natural enzymes found within vegetables and released into the juice by extraction provide most of the enzymes necessary for digestion and absorption. This allows the entire digestive system to approximate the rest of the water fast while still providing excellent energy and nutrition.

One of the key elements of vegetable juice fasts is their tendency to alkalinize the bloodstream, urine, and entire system of the faster. Over the years I have run thousands of urine tests on my participants—before the fast, during the bulking, and during the juice phase. Typically, the pre-fast urine is highly acidic and saturated with normal waste products, which can be measured as specific gravity of the urine. As the fast proceeds, the urine becomes less acidic and less concentrated. By the juice phase, most people have achieved an alkaline state, which is highly supportive of the body's normal waste elimination.

Because most noncellular wastes are stored in fat cells, bound to fatty acids, the breakdown of fats for fuel results in additional acid release into the bloodstream. Since we have a normal range of acidity and alkalinity in the human system, we cannot accept additional acid into a highly acidic system without negative consequences. By alkalinizing the system with a vegetable diet, we provide a buffer against an excessively acidic response to fatty acid conversion to fuel. It is not only a healthier state, but is also a much more enjoyable fasting experience for most people.

Fresh, nonpasteurized vegetable juices provide an abundant supply of antioxidants and enzymes, which are important to the cellular repair and rejuvenating properties of fasting. For most people this makes a much more energetic and effective fasting experience, which minimizes any negative aspects of mobilizing and eliminating toxins throughout the fast. Most people experience more energy and fewer bothersome symptoms than during their normal eating patterns while on the juice phase.

I have provided the basic juice recipes that I use for my fast, but you may choose to add additional vegetables into your juice program. Some of the traditional disease indications and juice choices are discussed in Chapter 3, pages 62–65. I have also included herbal considerations for specific and general disease states in this section. The addition of botanical and fungal extracts as powdered forms in solution, infusions (teas), and liquid forms are allowed but the use of capsules and tablets is discouraged during the liquid phase of the fast. Homeopathy, acupuncture, and hydrotherapy may also support the most productive experience of fasting and are discussed in the final chapter of this book.

The Enema

As mentioned earlier in the book, vegetable fasts require enemas for their optimal experience. I understand that the thought and act of enemas is too traumatic for a few individuals, and options for these situations are mentioned in the appendix. For most people the enema is not a bad experience and the recognizable benefits that it provides makes it an easy adjunct for most.

While there appears to be significant disagreement between many well-respected authors on fasting about whether enemas are needed or not, I have found these differences to be more associated with the type of fast than with the basic concept of enemas. I have found through personal experience that enemas are not typically required with pure water-only fasts or with the Master Cleanser program. Conversely, my experiences and those of my patients have shown that not doing enemas during a vegetable fast results in many negative occurrences. Fatigue, headaches, irritability, and even mild depression are common occurrences for people who go days on vegetable juices without doing enemas. It appears that the residual vegetable pulp found in vegetable juices coats the digestive tract, creating a barrier to the normal two-way traffic through the intestinal walls. As a result, toxins that are released into the bloodstream have less ability to dump (through the lymph system) into the colon and instead accumulate in the bloodstream, which leads to the unpleasant symptoms mentioned above. Many a stubborn or resistant faster has come in singing the praise of the enema from the dramatic improvements following their first experience.

How to Do an Enema

The first step is to buy an enema bag. These are readily available at most pharmacies and consist of a two-quart bag, hose and attachment, and generally two different speculums. The rectal speculum is the narrow one with one opening at the end. The speculum with the multiple small holes is a vaginal speculum and should not be used for the enema.

Use water that is close to body temperature. The tissues of the rectum and colon have similar heat tolerance to your mouth. While the solution can be significantly lower or higher than 98.6 degrees, the temperature influences the action of the enema. If the water is too cool, it will result in contraction of muscles making it difficult to leave the solution in for any length of time. Conversely, if the water is too warm, it will relax the colon and elimination of the fluid may be difficult and/or prolonged. You want to hold the enema solution for five to fifteen minutes, so you may adjust the temperature in following enemas to optimize the process. For example if you have difficulty voiding the solution at 98.6 degrees you may wish to use a cooler solution on following enemas. You do not need to be exact on the temperature. Typically the water temperature can be estimated by its sensation to the wrist, like testing the temperature of milk for a baby.

If you do an enema with water only, you will end up absorbing this water into your body due to the salt action of normal fluids. Water enemas are an excellent way to rehydrate, but counterproductive for the purposes of a fast. We want to pull from the body, thus opening the mineral and lymph drainage into the colon. (Recipes for enemas are provided on pages 116–118.)

When you have mixed your enema solution and filled the bag, you want to let gravity gently push the solution into the colon. There will be a plastic hanger in the enema kit, which you insert into the end of the bag and hang from a towel rack or about three to four feet above the floor. Use a natural ointment or products like Vaseline or KY Jelly to lubricate the speculum, and then insert it into the rectum while in a comfortable position. Figure 6.1 shows the most common position for enemas, but you can also lie on your side or back if these prove better for you. Once the speculum is inserted, release the clamp on the hose and allow as much solution to enter as is comfortable. You may not be able to take all two quarts in on the first day of juice but by day two or three this will be an easy amount to use.

Once you have taken in the solution, find a comfortable position and either gently massage the area of the large intestine or rest comfortably. After five to fifteen minutes, or sooner if necessary, void the solution into the toilet. It may take a couple of sittings to completely release the solution, so don't plan an enema in a tight schedule where you have to leave home and toilet soon after taking in the solution. Enema equipment should never be shared with others unless complete sterilization of equipment occurs after each use!

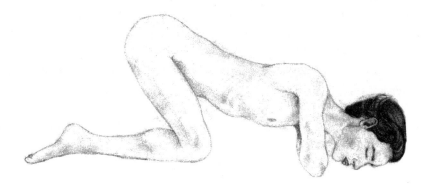

FIGURE 6.1 *Best Position for Administering an Enema*

Enema Solutions for a Five-Day Juice Phase

Here are recipes for enema solutions for each day of the juice fast. They can be used in any order except that the *Lactobacillus acidophilus* enema should be used on the last day.

Day One: Salt and Soda Enema

1 tablespoon sea salt
1 tablespoon baking soda
2 quarts of water

Dissolve sea salt and baking soda in water.

Day Two: Garlic–Epsom Salt Enema
This solution can be very purging.

3 cloves of garlic, chopped finely
2 quarts of water
2 tablespoons Epsom salt

Add garlic to water. Simmer for 5 minutes, then strain garlic out. Add Epsom salt. When cool, pour mixture into bag. Add water to fill bag and to reduce the temperature further.

Day Three or Four: Mae West's Coffee Enema
Do not do this enema late in the day, as caffeine may interfere with a restful sleep.

This enema has been recommended for patients with skin disease, hormone imbalances, chronic constipation, arthritis, and gout. This enema is NOT for patients with angina, heart disease, or uncontrolled high blood pressure. Patients with liver ailments and/or a history of past or present drug use (legal or illegal) should talk with a doctor about whether to use the Mae West.

This formula has been attributed to the late Mae West because it is said that she recognized the obvious relationship between colon congestion and skin health and appearance. Unwilling or unable to integrate the healthiest lifestyle and depending on her "Hollywood Beauty" reputation late into her career, she employed a weekly coffee enema as one of her beauty practices.

4 tablespoons ground coffee (not instant)
2 quarts of water
1 tablespoon sea salt
1 tablespoon baking soda

Use the ground coffee and water to make diluted coffee. (You can also do this by diluting 1 quart of standard drip coffee with 1 quart of water.) Add sea salt and baking soda. When cool enough, pour into bag.

Day Three or Four: Salt and Soda Enema
See recipe for Day One.

Last Day: *Lactobacillus Acidophilus* Enema
Do not use yogurt if you suspect a dairy allergy.

2 tablespoons yogurt, or 4 to 5 capsules acidophilus, or ⅛
teaspoon powdered acidophilus
2 quarts water

In water, mix yogurt OR empty 4 to 5 capsules of dry acidophilus OR add ⅛ teaspoon powdered acidophilus.

Additional Enema Options

Wheat Grass Enema

1 to 2 ounces fresh wheat grass juice (or green juice or chlorophyll)
2 quarts of water

Mix fresh wheat grass juice into water.

Vinegar Enema

2 tablespoons white vinegar
2 quarts of water

Mix white vinegar into water.

The enemas can be done any time of the day, except do not do the Mae West solution too late in the day because the caffeine will be partially absorbed and can definitely disturb sleep if done too late.

While there is no fixed order to the above recipes, the acidophilus enema logically falls on the final day of your juice program. It is important that you NOT do multiple coffee or Epsom salt enemas as these are more active solutions and will drain your energy if done frequently. If you choose to extend your juice phase, I recommend that you primarily repeat the basic salt and baking soda recipe through the extended program. You can repeat the coffee and Epsom salt formulas once each per additional week of juices.

The Colonic

A colonic is a type of colon-cleaning therapy that is typically administered by a qualified practitioner. It is used in the United States for both therapeutic and diagnostic purposes.

Colonic equipment continues to evolve with technological and medical advances. Unlike an enema, which uses a limited amount of water and generally cleans only the rectum, the colonic setup uses a system where water can be continuously inserted and released from the colon. This action allows a colonic treatment to remove wastes from the rectum all the way back to the ileocecal valve that connects the two intestines.

On a liquid fast a two-quart enema will also reach the ileocecal juncture and therefore provides an excellent support for the entire colon. Colonics, however, will still do a more thorough job of cleaning the colon than an enema, and you may choose to replace one or more daily enemas with a colonic. Licensure and practice of colonic therapy varies tremendously throughout the United States and other countries. Most important of all considerations is the issue of sterility, as many viral and microbial diseases can be transmitted if the practitioner does not follow appropriate sterilization procedures. Most practitioners should be able to provide safe equipment, but it is certainly your right to question a practitioner about the sterilization protocol.

Reintroducing Foods

The most important part of the fast is the appropriate reintroduction of foods. A long, successful fast that is concluded with a too-rapid reintroduction of complex foods may actually leave you more distressed than when you began. It is of the highest importance to reintroduce foods gradually with an appreciation of their relationship with the demands of digestion. The daily reintroduction program that follows includes a highly accurate protocol for determining food allergies and sensitivities.

Keep It Slow and Simple

Throughout a liquid fast, your entire digestive system has enjoyed a simpler, less-demanding state. Whether on a water or a juice fast, every cell and organ associated with digestion and normal elimination has had reduced demands and therefore has been in a resting and reparative state. It is logical that you would not want to go from this resting state to a meal of high fat and protein that immediately requires the entire effort of the digestive system for competent digestion. First foods after a fast should be those that require little effort to digest which would pretty much limit you to fruits and vegetables although some programs allow highly cooked cereal, like melba toast.

We would not engage in strenuous exercise without stretching and warming up, and the same sort of risk of strain or minor injury exists with the digestive system. Eating too dense a diet right after a fast will typically result in abdominal discomfort, bloating, and sometimes cramping and constipation. By slowly reintroducing foods, your digestive system should show the benefits of its rest and repair during the fast.

Sequence of Foods in Reintroduction

As described in Chapter 2, carbohydrates require the least energy and work for the process of digestion and absorption. Fats require more effort than carbohydrates, and proteins require the most work of all food categories. With this basic principle in mind, the logical sequence for reintroduction of foods is as follows.

- Fruits and nonstarchy vegetables
- Starchy vegetables like squash or yams; cereals, grains, and seeds
- Legumes and fats
- Proteins like nuts and meats

Cooking Time

In general, the more a food is cooked, the easier it is to digest. Cooking is an oxidative and predigestive process, which, while necessary for some foods, does result in destruction and loss of many micronutrients. We are always in that balance of how long to cook for maximum absorption, and how short to cook for maximum nutrition. Particularly in the vegetable kingdom, the more the crunch, the better the lunch.

Basic Guidelines for Reintroduction

My reintroduction program follows these basic guidelines, but some foods are introduced later than necessary as part of the allergy-testing protocol. In follow-up fasts, if you know you are not sensitive or allergic to these foods, they may be introduced in logical order with their associated food groups (for example, tomatoes and corn can enter on the first day of food for a five-day fast).

If you have extended the juice phase of this program, you may want to slow down the reintroduction process. If you have extended the phase to six or seven days, no change is necessary. For eight to fourteen days, I recommend you repeat the first day diet for a second day, minus the liver tonic, and then continue as outlined. If you have extended the fast longer than two weeks, the first day or two should only be soups and steamed vegetables, stewed and/or fresh fruit, broths, and juices followed by the two-day repeat of the reintroduction diet and normal conclusion. Guidelines for other fasting combinations are mentioned in the preceding chapter.

Allergies and Food Sensitivities

Food allergies and sensitivities are one of the most elusive, confusing, and frustrating areas of modern medicine. Not only are diagnostic procedures unable to distinguish between an allergy and a sensitivity, but the many tests available do not show the reliability necessary to accept their findings as accurate. In my experience the elimination protocol followed by food challenge has proven the most useful and accurate method to date.

This fasting program provides the foundation for informative and accurate self-determination of aggravating foods.

An allergy is a condition in which your immune system responds to a protein or hapton (a chemical that attaches to a protein, like penicillin) in a manner consistent with your antigen-antibody response to infection. When an allergic agent comes into contact with skin or respiratory tissue or is ingested, your immune system begins its release of immunoglobulins to fight off the invader. These are primarily of the Immunoglobulin G series (IGG) but may also include IGEs and IGMs. Most allergy tests that monitor immune response utilize the specific IGG response to detect your response. Hyperreactivity, including anaphylactic response, is an extreme phase of allergy and will not be covered in this text.

Food sensitivities also activate a similar immune response, but unlike true allergies, these are developed or acquired over time with incomplete digestion. Sensitivities can be reversed if the underlying causes of poor digestion are addressed. True allergies cannot be reversed, although desensitization is possible. Clinically and subjectively, the symptoms and clinical changes of sensitivities and allergies are identical. It is only after elimination and improvement of digestive function that the sensitivity can be distinguished from the allergen. I have had innumerable patients become able to safely and healthfully consume foods for which they previously showed allergic responses.

I was long ago taught that allergy and addiction were synonymous terms for many situations. While this seems contrary to the natural order of the body, it is understandable when you look at what is happening at the microscopic and cellular level. Proteins are typically of enormous microscopic structure, and as outlined in Chapter 2, they require a complex sequence of acids and enzymes in order to be reduced to absorbable nutrients called peptides. In the wall of the intestines, these peptides are further reduced into individual amino acids, which are the desired forms for healthy digestion. When we lack the enzymes to competently digest foods, or have an inflammatory condition that leads to incomplete digestion, large protein structures are absorbed into the bloodstream. This macro-absorption can occur through two methods, either through giant cells in the gut or through a process of hyper-permeability of inflamed tissues. Either way, incompletely digested proteins enter the bloodstream and begin the reactive immune response.

In the bloodstream and also at the contact tissues of the gut, your white blood cells encounter these large structures. When your cells recognize the structures as not being usable nutrients and not being of your own creation, they call out for help from other cells to fight off this invader. This begins the complex cycle of T-cell regulation, which results in the release of specific immunoglobulins to attack these invaders. Unlike bacteria, fungi, viruses, and parasites, which will multiply in number, these undigested proteins are reduced in number by the liver, so when the immunoglobulins arrive at the scene there is reduced substrate for them to act upon. Like the story of the boy who cried wolf, this leaves a confused environment with the potential for your immune system to turn upon your own tissue—an autoimmune response. I have had numerous cases of autoimmune conditions, arthritis, and other clinically diagnosed conditions completely disappear when food allergens have been removed. One theorized solution for this confusion is to keep eating the aggravating foods, thereby guaranteeing that there will be an enemy for the immunoglobulins to attack. Hence, allergy can equal addiction. Any time a patient brings me a diet diary with a particular food appearing eighteen to twenty-one meals per week, I am nearly convinced that either that food is an allergen or that a developed sensitivity exists.

If you are allergic to a food that you rarely eat, you immediately recognize the immune response, and you are likely not to eat that food again. When that food is a mainstay of your diet, its ingestion is accompanied by preexisting immunoglobulins so the response is more like what you feel when you go from fifty to fifty-five mph on the freeway, or nearly unnoticeable. It is only when you have gone many days without that food that you return to the zero to fifty mph sensation that allows detection of the problem. Five or more days on juices or a hypoallergenic diet will guarantee an accurate detection environment.

Allergic responses are numerous and quite varied. They include virtually all the symptoms that you experience with an infection, as your unpleasant sensations of illness are almost entirely the symptoms of immune response and not microbial action. These symptoms include:

- Increased or rapid pulse
- Shortness of breath
- Rashes or itchy skin
- Light-headedness
- Fatigue
- Heart palpitations
- Stiffness or achy joints and muscles
- Nausea and or diarrhea
- Nasal drainage, stuffiness, or sneezing
- Mood swings (depression, anxiety, and irritability)
- Headaches and migraines
- Gas and or bloating

When you eat a frequently consumed food, these symptoms are of a vague and chronic nature. When you introduce potential allergens following this juice fast, the symptoms are generally unmistakable. If they are minor, then the sensitivity is typically of a minor nature and reduction or rotation of these foods may well be adequate to establish a healthy relationship. Pulse-rate increases after a fast are significant and often involve an increase of more than 50 percent. (If resting rate is 60 beats per minute, or bpm, allergic reaction may be 90–120 bpm for the short time following consumption.)

I have found this post-fasting food challenge to be exceptionally accurate and useful for my patients. There have been many significant improvements in my patients' health with the removal or rotation of aggravating foods. The following reintroduction plan includes the most common foods that show up as allergens (and they are boldfaced). These include dairy, eggs, potatoes, wheat, soy, peanuts, corn, tomatoes, and citrus fruits (especially oranges). If you suspect another food or foods to be a problem, please isolate these foods during your reintroduction as they too can be accurately tested.

To check for sensitivity to a food, ingest it alone or with foods to which you know you are not sensitive. During the reintroduction, bold-faced foods should not be introduced at the same meal, since both are common allergens. For example, on day two of the reintroduction, you should add yogurt to one meal, and tomatoes to another. Remember that there are two possible reactions to dairy, the first being to the proteins and the second, called lactose intolerance, to the lactose or sugar in milk. Yogurt is a form of dairy where the lactose is predigested, and if you react to yogurt, that means a protein-based reactivity and all dairy products are a problem. If you don't react to yogurt, but do react to noncultured dairy such as milk or cheese, then you probably have a lactose intolerance and can often safely consume dairy with the support of lactase enzymes available at health foods stores and pharmacies.

Outside of severe reactions, such as allergic asthma, your respiratory function is partially voluntary and a difficult indicator of response. The pulse is entirely out of most people's conscious response, so it can serve you very well as a testing tool. To check your pulse response, check your pulse rate immediately before ingesting a boldfaced food. Check it again at fifteen, thirty, and sixty minutes following ingestion of this food. An elevated response of 50 percent or more suggests a clear sensitivity or allergy. It is possible to be allergic to a food without it influencing your heart rate, so be sure to observe all the symptom changes mentioned above. Rarely will someone have all the symptom changes noted, and typically the areas of response will parallel preexisting chronic concerns.

The Reintroduction Diet

It's important to remember that the key to a successful fast is coming out of it slowly!

Day One

The first day that you reintroduce solid foods into your diet begins with the liver flush tonic as prescribed on page 105 of this chapter. Unlike the pre-fast diet, the liver tonic is not followed by fiber and herbal laxatives but is taken one time only to prepare your digestive system, liver, and gall bladder for the addition of normal fats into the diet.

Day One is intended not to have any potential allergens included in your foods, but as you may note, citrus is a component of the liver tonic, so watch for any reactions to this drink. Foods allowed on the first day include only those that require a minimum of digestive effort. They are pretty much limited to the fruit and vegetable kingdoms, but they exclude common allergens in these groups such as corn, tomatoes, and potatoes. Also excluded from this category of minimal digestive effort are the hard squashes, yams, and sweet potatoes. The vegetables and fruits can be prepared as homemade soups (vegetables only, no meat or soy base), salads, steamed vegetables, juices, smoothies, and teas. There is no set amount of food that you must eat as you reintroduce foods. Remember that optimal digestion includes chewing your foods well, both to increase access to the nutrients by your enzymes and to stimulate the important enzyme release of the glands of the mouth.

As I've explained earlier, juice fasting does not lower your metabolism, so the yo-yo phenomenon of starvation diets and other fad programs is not to be expected. The juice fast as I've employed it over the years has resulted in great benefits including optimizing weight so that both under- and overweight people move to a more ideal normal weight. Your digestive system has had a period of resting and repair and in all probability is more efficient than in the recent past, so the same number of calories in the mouth may end up being more calories delivered into the bloodstream. It is important to eat slowly and allow your body to acclimate to this improved functioning.

Day Two

the homemade soups, vegetable and fruit salads, steamed :es, smoothies, and teas, Day Two adds millet (the most r common cereal grain families), **yogurt**, and **tomatoes**. foods are the first of the common allergens and should be arately, at least one hour apart. There are no further liver tonics after Day One and there is no requirement that you eat everything on the allowable list. Each day opens up to more allowable choices of foods but only the boldfaced foods are specifically suggested as important inclusions.

If a boldfaced food or any other foods on these lists are foods that you avoid, it is not necessary to eat them. If you don't eat a food because you suspect, rather than know, that you are allergic or sensitive to it, you may want to eat it once just to confirm or refute your suspicions.

Day Three

On the third day of food reintroduction, you are allowed to add barley, yams, sweet potatoes, winter squash, **potatoes**, and **citrus fruits**. For the last two foods, a serving of one to two tablespoons is adequate for testing purposes. You are still able to include any of the foods allowed on preceding days as is true throughout the reintroduction diet.

Day Four

On Day Four your list of acceptable foods expands to include brown rice, legumes (**peanuts** and **soy**), and **eggs**. The increased sense of taste and smell that comes with fasting continues throughout the reintroduction. This is a great time to find satisfaction and enjoyment from whole foods, and a great time to try new foods as you establish a healthier diet.

Day Five

This is the day that the most common American allergen, **wheat**, is added. Please test with a whole-wheat product, as opposed to processed wheat, which is both less nutritious and has much less protein content for allergy testing. For some people who have mild sensitivities to wheat, the processed form may actually do less insult, from an allergic standpoint, and a rotation diet might well include this form in spite of its obvious nutritional limitations. You can also add other grains (rye, oats, triticale, **corn**), and **dairy** products (cheese), excluding foods you've already established a sensitivity or allergy to.

If you had a reaction to yogurt on Day Two, it is unnecessary to test other dairy products because you will also be sensitive to them. There are times when goat or nonbovine (not from cattle) products may be well tolerated, so if you reacted to cow's yogurt, you may want to try feta or other goat-derived dairy products as a substitute.

Day Six

This is the final scheduled day of reintroduction of solid foods. On this day we add the most complex digestive demands with such foods as meats, nuts (**walnuts**), and supplemental **yeast**, such as nutritional yeast, baker's yeast, and brewer's yeast. Again, you do not need to add or test foods that are not part of your normal diet.

You have hopefully enjoyed the expanded varieties of whole foods, which by the final day include homemade soups, fruit and vegetable salads, steamed vegetables, smoothies, juices and teas, millet, **yogurt**, **tomatoes**, barley, yams and sweet potatoes, **potatoes**, winter squash, **citrus fruits**, brown rice, legumes (**peanuts, soy**), **eggs, wheat products** and other grains (rye, oats, triticale, **corn**), **dairy products**, meats, nuts (**walnuts**), and supplemental **yeast**. The choices you make after Day Six are up to you. You will have done a great service to your body, mind, and spirit—and may well want to continue to honor them with more conscious consumption as you continue to explore the relationships between your diet and your health.

If you have multiple reactions to foods in the first few days of the reintroduction, you may not get good feedback as the reintroduction continues. If you only have a few reactive experiences, your food challenges on Day Six will still be quite informative.

Coffee, alcohol, processed foods, and foods with additives, preservatives, and other added sugars or chemicals should not be included in your reintroduction diet. Please aim for moderation or avoidance of these foods as much as possible in your day-to-day practices.

Interpreting Allergic Responses

The information that you get from your reintroduction of foods can help you achieve your optimal diet. If you are allergic or sensitive to a given food, then the costs of eating this food often outweigh the benefits of the nutrition found within. Without identification, you may continue to eat these foods and feel sluggish, catch more colds, have more digestive upset, experience chronic muscle ache or stiffness, or present more severe allergic symptoms like chronic sinusitis or rashes. You may receive the diagnosis of gastroenteritis, depression, fibromyalgia, middle-ear infections (otitis media), hypoglycemia, respiratory infections, or other conditions that are mimicked by your allergic responses. Failure of these conditions to respond to medical intervention may speak to their allergic origin. By isolating and eliminating specific food allergies or sensitivities, you may be on your way to discovering the mysterious cause of these conditions from a more complete, effective, and logical approach.

If you have monitored your reintroduction of specific foods and watched for the heightened responses of a hypoallergenic fast, you should have an understanding of how severe your allergy or sensitivity is. If you have dramatic increases in pulse rate, significant changes in respiration, or severe responses as noted in the above text, you should consider complete elimination of the food from your diet.

Allergy or Sensitivity?

As has been discussed, you may be able to reverse a sensitivity, but never a true allergen. To determine the difference between allergen and sensitivity, keep a food out of your diet for two to three months as you work to improve your digestive function and ecology. If, upon reintroduction, you still react strongly, you probably need to consider not eating that food because it more likely is a true allergen and not an acquired sensitivity.

Food Rotation

If your response to a given food is mild, then the concept of food rotation is probably adequate to maintain a healthful relationship with these foods. This simply means that you don't eat this food every meal or even every day. Frequency, per week, is determined again by the severity of these lesser responses. Typically, twice per week is a safe rotation of suspicious foods. In general it is good to rotate foods and seek out the maximum variety in your diet.

7

Simply Nutritious

If you believe in the creation theory, you should believe that the Creator placed upon the earth all foods necessary for ideal health. If you believe in the theory of evolution, then you must hold that your survival and health is dependent on your evolved diet. Either way, you must seriously question your significant departure from your natural nutritional resources.

Basic Concepts in Nutrition

I have always found nutrition to be a simple science. I can credit my mother and father for providing a good foundation in basic nutrition. They combined common sense, farm upbringings, personal responsibility, and scientific inquiry in my childhood experience and thus into my daily diet. We rarely had processed foods, always had ample vegetables and a salad at dinner, and an abundance of whole cereals, legumes, and other healthy, inexpensive items. Foods that we grew, picked, or bought, we canned ourselves, thereby avoiding the huge onslaught of artificial chemicals and preservatives that entered the American food chain during my childhood.

Science, math, and athletics were my focus and passions as a child. Like any favored area of study and practice, these fields have continued to interest me throughout my life and therefore are rather easy subjects for me to observe and understand. My criticism of nutritional science comes not from disrespect, but from knowledge of its frequent misinterpretations. Scientific investigation itself is a very valuable element of our present and future well-being. Until research is removed from the single-nutrient disease investigation that is the nature of medical science—and until it is removed from the economic interests involved—the scientific study of disease and nutrition cannot provide a working model that can clearly serve the general public. Until our understanding of nutrition from the microscopic perspective is much more complete, the constant revelations of new scientific facts will often lead to more confusion instead of understanding. I will provide some of the simple concepts from which a more useful understanding of diet and nutrition can be utilized on a personal level.

One of the most basic concepts in nutrition is the calorie. This word is rooted in the Latin term *calor*, or heat, and truly, a food calorie is the measurement of how much thermal heat is generated when one gram of food is incinerated in a test tube. We think of calories as a human or living relationship with the fuel of foods, as well as nutritional worth. This is a truly erroneous concept because we are much more than a laboratory test tube and match. Calories of foods do not represent true fuel for the body because there is an immense variation in your digestive efficiency with different foods. As discussed in Chapter 2, it takes much longer and requires more work by the digestive system to digest and absorb proteins than to digest fats or sugars. According to modern physiology, it takes about 100 calories of work to digest 100 calories of protein. Conversely, it only takes about 5 calories of work to digest 100 calories of simple refined sugars. In part, this is why the high-protein diet is a lean or weight-loss type of diet. You simply have to get your fuel energy from nonprotein sources. And if you avoid additional sugars or fats, you tap into reserve energy supplies, or fat cells—and lose weight.

Foods are generally broken down into three categories: proteins, fats, and carbohydrates or sugars. Each of these three categories is further divided into subcategories. For proteins, we recognize the essential amino acids, meaning it is essential that we consume these specific proteins in adequate amounts to maintain health, and nonessential amino acids that make up the rest of the proteins in our diets. Similarly, fats are broken down into the two very important essential fats, linoleic and linolenic acids (some authors add arachidonic acid) and nonessential fats. Food-related fats are divided into saturated (animal source), monosaturated such as olive oil, and polyunsaturated (which includes the essential fats). Carbohydrates or sugars are generally divided into simple and complex. Simple sugars include lactose from milk, fructose from fruits, glucose and other related members that we recognize as sweet. Complex carbohydrates are the much larger starchy sugars from cereals, grains, legumes, squash, and other vegetables. Rarely are whole foods pure protein or pure fat, but contain combinations of these basic food structures.

When you eat an abundance of whole, minimally processed vegetables, cereals, grains, and fruits, you are getting an equal abundance of fiber and water, two very important components of your diet. When you eat a diet of highly refined foods, these two normal components of foods become inadequate and this results in a negative impact on the body and the status of your health. You must have adequate fiber to effectively carry out your digestive wastes, and you must have adequate water, or hydration, to aid the work of fiber, support liver and kidney function, and promote cellular health. *The Diseases of Women, Their Causes and Cure*, written in 1858, contains the following advice: "White bread is neither so nourishing, nor so wholesome as that with bran in it, though a mistaken notion to the contrary prevails."[1] The author continues to explain how fiber aids elimination and prevents diseases of the colon and liver. It took the FDA nearly 120 years to acknowledge the common-sense relationship between fiber and disease that has been evident to doctors in the field since the inception of processed foods in the 1800s.

Processing of foods, which involves changing the basic makeup of the food, has cost us dearly over the past two hundred years. Refining foods often removes or decreases the content of essential fats, fiber, vitamins, and enzymes. This is also true of overcooking of foods, which is an oxidative process that can significantly reduce the micronutrient content of whole foods.

In 1995 I did field research on natural medicine and the delivery of medical care in Chile. I am always interested in how traditional and conventional medicine blend into other cultures and how available medical care is to the general population. I had the wonderful opportunity to meet and talk at length with Pedro Silva, M.D., Homeopath, and what the South Americans call a "Naturista." Dr. Silva has authored many books on diet, herbal medicine, and vegetarian approach to nutrition. In our conversations he provided his observations on diet change and disease in Chile, which I am relating here.

In the late 1980s two cases of cholera were diagnosed in Santiago, Chile. The military government, fearing a cholera outbreak, initiated their first public education campaign since the time of democratic rule in the early 1970s. They told people to cook all vegetables and foods until they were soft and thoroughly cooked in order to kill any disease-causing bacteria. What was witnessed in Dr. Silva's eyes, and in the health of his patients, was the unprecedented emergence of Western diseases, including cancer, heart disease, and diabetes—this in a society that had maintained good health for the many decades before. Certainly, cholera outbreaks need to be controlled, but thousands of deaths and the tremendous worsening of health of the general population as witnessed in Chile is an unnecessary price for the prevention of food-borne disease. Dr. Silva clearly felt the overcooking of essential nutrients was the sole cause of their Western disease patterns.

We have seen the Western diet take its toll as people relocate to Western nations and as the Western approach to diet moves into other countries. When traveling in Asia and South America I see obesity in tourists from America and Europe and not in the general populations. Concepts such as a genetic cause of obesity can only be defended by scientists who spend time in the laboratory and not in the real world. There may be genetic factors in how someone responds to the inadequate diet of modern times, but most obesity and disease is far more related to our modern diet than any genetic predisposition.

We can play the nutrition games of fad diets and science by counting and balancing calories, fats, proteins, and carbohydrates and by guaranteeing adequate fiber, vitamins, and minerals, and yet be far from ideal health and nutrition. Roger Williams, M.D., in his book *Nutrition Against Disease*, wrote eloquently about the limitations of science in being able to isolate all-important nutrients in our foods. He coined the term *biochemical individuality* as he recognized that among his genetically identical laboratory rats, there existed up to a twenty-fold difference in minimum requirements of protein intake to prevent known protein-related diseases. We are far from identical laboratory humans, and the establishment of nutritional requirements would logically be even more diverse in us than in Williams's animals.

Dr. Williams was the first person to identify, isolate, and synthesize pantothenic acid, and he also identified and named folic acid. His brother, R. R. Williams, is credited with initiating the enrichment practice in processed foods in 1941. Forty years later, Dr. Williams called enrichment a complete fraud. While he felt that his brother's selection of the four initial nutrients that he had identified as being depleted by processing was a logical first enrichment step, the list of nutrients removed through processing had grown tremendously. In spite of the new knowledge, enriched flour still included only potassium, iron, riboflavin, and niacin as replacement nutrients. The fraud was that the term *enriched* suggests an improved product, whereas enrichment practices clearly result in foods that are deficient in their original nutritional content.

We need continued study of the micronutrient levels of our foods, knowing that our information is and will remain far from complete.

Observations of diet and the health status of society remain invaluable to creating a workable foundation of nutritional science. History reminds us that it was Japanese doctors in the late 1800s who noted that few prisoners got beriberi or pellagra while these diseases were rampant in the general population. Observations of societal patterns led these doctors to question widely held misconceptions about the cause of these diseases. While the popular germ theory of Pasteur led medicine to believe that these diseases must be caused by a microbial infection, events soon led to a different understanding.

In 1886 Dutch physician Eijkman was sent to Java to isolate the microbial cause of beriberi. While Eijkman rejected the Japanese theory that beriberi was somehow related to a nutritional deficiency, his scientific objectivity changed his mind. After twenty years of study, he too came to believe beriberi to be of nutritional origin. His study and subsequent isolation of vitamin B earned him the Nobel Prize in Medicine in the 1930s. Shortly after Eijkman publicly supported the nutritional deficiency theory of beriberi, Casimir Funk, a Polish-born biochemist, proposed the *vitamine theory* of disease. He not only proposed that deficiency of some vital amino acid causes beriberi but that pellagra, rickets, and scurvy were also of nutritional origin. With the later discovery that some vitamins like vitamin C were not protein-based amino acids, the word *vitamin* emerged.

Integration of the *vitamine theory* into natural medicine began as early as 1916 when J. H. Kellogg, M.D., in his book *Colon Hygiene*, spoke of the vitamin content of whole foods. Kellogg, who is considered one of the founders of Naturopathic Medicine, advocated an ovo-lacto vegetarian approach to diet. He noted the need for high-fiber, vitamin-rich whole fruits and vegetables for healthy digestive function and general health. His development of "Corn Flakes" as an additive-free, whole-grain food honored his written belief that white flour and processed foods contribute to or were responsible for most diseases. The understanding of optimum nutritional needs is far from complete, but it has strongly influenced our understanding of food as more than protein, fat, sugar, and starch.

The Four Basic Truths of Ideal Nutrition

Understanding that biochemical individuality exists, that our knowledge of micronutrients is far from complete, and that different whole foods contain different important nutrients, we can see a simpler path to ideal nutrition. Along this path there are four basic truths:

- Whole and organic foods are the best.
- Variety is very important.
- Minimize the processing and cooking of your foods.
- Pay attention to your individual response to foods.

Organic Versus Nonorganic Foods

Government agencies and scientific communities often insist that organic foods are not inherently better than nonorganic foods; their arguments are hollow and without merit. Let us review some of the important differences between organic and nonorganic foods.

The term *organic* when applied to agriculture implies the production and growth of foods without the use of synthetic fertilizers, pesticides, fungicides, or other synthetic chemical treatment. Different governments and municipalities define organic products by their own standards. In the United States the term organic generally means that the nonsynthetic practice has continued at least five years in the same soil. Those farms initially integrating organic methods are referred to as transitional organic because chemical residues are often found for at least five years in the soil and therefore in the produce grown in that soil. Organic is more than just the absence of pesticides and synthetic chemicals. It is, logically, a more complete and nutritional food product.

With the USDA and the FDA primarily concerned with the presence or absence of these nonorganic chemical residues, their evaluation of nutritional equality is so limited as to be scientifically flawed and without merit. There are commonly accepted scientific principles and findings that support this criticism. Even though people claim to be able to taste the difference between organic produce and commercial equivalents, this is considered irrelevant. Regardless of how consistently people may taste or feel the difference, organic and nonorganic are considered equivalent from a nutritional standpoint. The true differences are easy to identify from a conceptual standpoint, but they are more difficult to measure in common practice.

The use of synthetic fertilizers involves the limited replacement of only three soil minerals: potassium, nitrogen, and phosphorus. These nutrients have proven themselves as potent stimulators of plant growth and crop production, not as maintainers of complete nutritional composition. The question remains: what is it that we are yielding with this limited soil replacement?

Our earth's soils are naturally filled with a multitude of valuable trace minerals. These minerals continue to be replaced by the trace minerals found in the breakdown of organic vegetation. An abundance of scientific studies show an inverse relationship with selenium levels in soil and hence the food content of selenium, an important trace mineral, and the incidence of cancer. In other words, the less naturally occurring selenium in the diet, the greater the incidence of many forms of cancer. Other important trace minerals found in foods and required by humans, through dietary or supplemental nutrition, include zinc (immune function, digestive function, cell division, neuro-processing), chromium (insulin function, diabetes), magnesium, calcium, and manganese, to name just a few. Doctors would never recommend that we provide our children with only three minerals and not worry about all the others. We know that without calcium, we could not develop normal bones. Without iodine, we could not manufacture thyroid hormone to regulate normal metabolic function. The relationship of minerals and trace minerals with normal human function is well documented in any general nutrition text, yet we somehow maintain that plants have no need or use for their historical soil nutrition if provided synthetic alternatives.

The FDA and USDA do not consider trace mineral equivalence between organic and nonorganic foods. Therefore, no difference exists, end of story. What a sad commentary, especially for those who appreciate true scientific methodology. We are constantly discovering new antioxidants, enzymes, and other phytonutrients in our foods, but again, we are far from a complete list. The very real question exists: will we complete this list before our food and soil have been so altered that we no longer have a complete model of study?

An alarming difference between organic and nonorganic agriculture is their impact on the soil itself. Organic methods of agriculture increase or maintain topsoil, whereas commercial methods result in significant loss of topsoil. More importantly, petrochemical fertilizers and a wide number of commonly used pesticides and fungicides significantly damage the soil organisms that plants depend on for absorption of soil nutrients. Much like the human condition of dysbiosis discussed in Chapter 2, this alteration of soil microflora has an unquestioned negative impact on plant life. We become ever more dependent upon the use of pesticides, fungicides, and other chemical intervention as we have destroyed the long-standing balance of our soil, its friendly microbes, and the plant kingdom.

The notion that nonorganic produce is equal to organic produce is a difficult argument to believe. The recent linkage of pesticide intake by humans and increased rates of hormonal cancers, like breast cancer, is of major concern. The presentation of a wide array of Western, chronic diseases may never be closely linked to our agricultural practices, but the long-standing disinterest by most governmental agencies in these logical relationships weakens our trust in their overall concern for the public welfare.

Genetically Modified Foods

One final area of modern changes to our dietary choices needs to be discussed. Genetically modified organisms (GMOs) began entering the human diet in the early 1990s. Just as in the case of organic versus nonorganic foods, the FDA currently maintains that this new science is safe and that genetically modified foods are identical to existing foods. Proponents of this new technology maintain that it is no different from past techniques of hybridization of plants, and that the growing public suspicions and criticisms are alarmist and unfounded. Everyone is entitled to his or her own opinion, however I maintain that there is no complete scientific evidence of safety, and that this ongoing human and planetary experiment has the potential of truly dire consequences. The past mistakes of the FDA in providing consumer confidence in such drugs as acutane, DES, and alar may be dwarfed by the potential magnitude of harm resulting from genetic modification.

It is possible that genetic modification may prove beneficial in the long run. But I believe that it is highly unlikely that more good than harm will come. I choose to do everything in my power to exclude these new foods from my family's diet. The true proof of safety, the human experiment, will take decades to conclude, unless instances of acute harm from GMOs to our population force a major revision of policy. It is critical that the FDA allow specific labeling of non-GMOs, so that our public is empowered and enabled to make its own personal dietary choices. In the absence of this appropriate labeling, it is even more important to use organic products or ask each company for documentation of non-GMO ingredients.

The prevailing logic behind the development of GMOs is that we can more quickly produce new plant strains that will provide equal or better nutrition, will be more resistant to infestation, and will provide greater crop yields. These are certainly admirable goals, and if "the end justifies the means" is what matters in science and ethics, then this experiment might be justified. The current track record of GMOs just doesn't appear headed toward an end to hunger or a safer, more nutritious food industry.

Questions and concerns about GMOs are many. Before elaborating on these issues, it is important to understand what GMOs are and how this technology differs from historical methods of hybridization.

The selective breeding and cross-pollination of plant species dates back thousands of years. The Chinese have written documentation about selective cultivation of the peony nearly five thousand years ago. We have selectively chosen qualities in domestic animals and encouraged the selective breeding of the "best" traits. This has resulted in chickens that lay more eggs, cows that produce more milk, and dogs that exhibit better-trained qualities. Equally, inbreeding has occasionally worked to the contrary and resulted in significant losses in overall health or quality.

In our agricultural past, we have always stayed within the same species of animals or plants, depending upon their reproductive compatibility when crossbreeding. Genetic modification is absolutely a different process, and comparisons between GMOs and traditional hybridization are unfounded, ingenuine, and potentially dishonest.

I have visited facilities that do genetic engineering. I have interviewed the genetic scientists and spoken to FDA officials about the technology. I have not been impressed with the arguments from any of the players. The discussions have been of such limited scope that true evaluation of impact is beyond their review and beyond current knowledge. Let's look at the process of genetic modification.

The Process of Genetic Modification

One of the most prevalent techniques of genetic modification is the use of "benign" viruses to invade a plant's DNA and carry a new encrypted program into the plant's genetic memory. What is carried into the new plant by the viruses can be virtually any genetic information and may include genetic codes from other species of plants or from animals or other life forms such as fungi or bacteria. Pesticide production, resistance to frost or dehydration, and any biologic process of DNA-based life can theoretically be encrypted into the original DNA. Where the virus places the new information is basically a random event. The new seed, or what grows, is the final determinant of success or failure. What has been removed from the plant's genetic code with this insertion is often unknown and ultimately considered inconsequential. If the new product looks like, tastes like, and has similar fat, protein, sugar, fiber, and water content as the original, it is considered identical.

No comprehensive evaluation of the complete micronutrient content of GMOs is required or possible at the present time.

Questions About GMOs

Unanswered questions about GMOs include:

- Will some religious practices be compromised by the inclusion of animal genes into vegetable products?
- Will the pollens of these new plants harm the existing ecology? There exists some evidence that pollens have already been linked to harming monarch butterflies and to sterilizing native seeds of adjoining crops.
- Since GMOs are predominantly sterile, meaning that farmers have to continually buy new seeds, will this harm small farmers in third world nations? Will it allow seed access to be used as a leverage for special interests?
- Will pesticides that are produced internally by plants prove harmful to individuals or whole populations?
- Will we lose important nutrients from our historical food supplies?
- Will insertion of new DNA result in allergic sensitivity by individuals? As an added insult, without labeling, someone who knows that he or she is allergic to a specific food may not realize that another food now contains that same allergen.
- Will the encryption viruses always be absent from the food, and if not, might they have the potential to alter human DNA expression?

With so many unanswerable questions, how can we be confident that these new foods are 100 percent safe? Despite claims of equivalence and safety, many people are highly skeptical of this technology. It is up to you to decide whether you perceive these foods as safe enough for you to participate in this human and planetary experiment.

Micronutrients

The term *micronutrient* came to us in the twentieth century. It is a self-explanatory word in that it literally means "small foods," or those substances found in foods that we need in small or microscopic portions. Macronutrients make up the majority of the substance of our diet and include our fuel, materials of cellular and tissue structure, and eliminatory materials of fiber and water. These are the basic constituents of food or calories—proteins, fats, and carbohydrates and the essential but indigestible fiber.

Micronutrients include essential fats, essential amino acids, vitamins, minerals, and enzymes as well as an ever-growing list of phytonutrients and fungal nutrients. The concept of micronutrients goes back to the nineteenth century when doctors theorized that some unknown factor(s) existed in foods, which in dietary adequacy prevented, and in absence led to, the diseases scurvy, beriberi, and pellagra. These three factors were later recognized as vitamins C, B_1, and B_2. Even earlier in medical history, the Roman physician Galen found that minerals, as cremated ash, were found in all human and animal tissues. This led to a broader understanding of human nutrition as well as inserting the use of minerals and metals in the Western model of medicine.

The need for vitamins and minerals in our diet is well established. The levels of specific nutrients required to avoid single-nutrient–related diseases is fairly consistent within medicine, but the level of micronutrients necessary for optimal health varies widely from source to source. Our list of required vitamins has expanded from the original dietary factors theorized in the late 1800s to dozens of vitamins and hundreds of important micronutrients. It is clear that we don't have a complete list of all human required nutrients. There is also a large body of research and evidence to suggest that many disease conditions are reduced in frequency and severity with nonvitamin, nonmineral factors found in our diet. This evidence is not limited to the early live enzyme research of Dr. William Pottinger, but his body of research alone places vegetable enzymes into the category of required nutrients. Dr. Pottinger, working with tens of thousands of laboratory cats, found that the addition of fresh, diced vegetables in his cat feed significantly reduced most chronic diseases. Current science should seriously question the reluctance of medicine to admit that our agricultural and dietary practices are significant contributors to many, if not most, of our Western disease and health care costs.

I wrote earlier about the concept of biochemical individuality, as discovered by Dr. Roger Williams. Many traditional as well as contemporary sources have also based their nutritional recommendations upon individual characteristics. The more familiar systems include the Ayurvedic classification of four body types and contemporary theories such as the simple division by blood types in *Eat Right 4 Your Type* by Dr. Peter D'Adamo. Physicians and researchers have noted different responses to the same diet, based upon observable or measurable differences within the human population. It is clear that biochemical individuality does exist regarding exact amounts of nutrients required to prevent and resist disease. It is also clear that we do not have current technology or science to exactly quantify an individual's optimal needs of a given micronutrient. Your own sense of wellness and your own response to your foods as well as clinical and laboratory measurements of various health parameters remain your best roadmap to your own nutritional needs.

I have no confidence that any one dietary theory adequately deals with the individual variations of nutritional needs. Not only does biochemical individuality exist, but also there are a number of other factors that influence what is the healthiest diet for any given person. Digestive function, intestinal microflora, allergies, and food sensitivities are areas of individual variability. Personal, familial, and social relationships with food also exist. Just because a food or dish has measurable nutritional value does not mean that we will enjoy eating it or maintain it as a regular part of our diet. Not only do pleasurable smells and tastes of food increase your digestive enzymes and immune function, but also they evoke a whole array of personal responses. For long-term dietary choices, it is important that you incorporate an approach that satisfies your lifestyle and taste pleasures as well as your nutritional needs. Short-term dietary changes rarely produce long-term benefit.

With an understanding that neither I nor any author can name all the necessary micronutrients or provide exact individual amounts of known micronutrients needed for optimal health, I provide the following brief review of important nutrients in the human diet.

Essential Fatty Acids

I know of no area of nutrition where so much misinformation and therefore public confusion exists as in the discussion of fats and oils. Compounding this problem is the widely held belief that dietary fat is strongly related to the prevention or development of many Western diseases. I believe this common belief is well founded but that the magnitude of these disease relationships is significantly underappreciated by contemporary medicine. I feel that the destruction of water soluble vitamins, enzymes, and essential fats in modern preparation and processing of vegetables and the substantial reduction in consumption of essential fats are the two most detrimental changes of modern diet. Increasing your intake of fresh minimally cooked or raw vegetable and seeds and of essential fats is a critical step to a healthier society.

Essential fatty acids (EFAs) are defined as specific fats that humans must consume in a structurally intact form to live and to thrive. There are two generally recognized essential fats. These are linoleic and linolenic acids. They are what we call omega-3 and omega-6 fats, which means in chemical nomenclature that there is a carbon double-bond on the third or sixth carbon atom of a given fat molecule. The human system can manufacture double bonds anywhere on a fat molecule from the seventh carbon on out. Many important chemicals of human physiology require third and sixth carbon double-bonding, so we must consume these oils in our diet or as supplements.

A critical part of the use of essential fats is dependent upon the structural integrity of these oils. Udo Erasmus, in his book *Fats and Oils*, provides some of the best understanding of essential fats and general fat relationships with disease. He furthers his discussion on these relationships in his second book, *Fats That Heal, Fats That Kill*. In his work he discusses how these two fats are universally produced within the plant kingdom as an essential ingredient of photosynthesis. They are very responsive to levels of heat or ultraviolet light, consistent with the ranges of normal sunlight. This means that they are easily destroyed by heat extraction, hydrogenation, excessive cooking, or prolonged exposure to UV light. This destruction not only results in reduced nutrition, but can also result in toxic fat by-products called trans fatty acids.

In nature, meaning within the cells of plants, double bonds of linoleic and linolenic acids are always found in the cis formation. In what chemistry calls the stereochemistry of molecules, this simply means that in a carbon double bond, the next adjoining carbons are positioned so that they bend toward each other and not away from each other as is true of trans fatty acids. Like flipping a coin, in nonplant processing of fats, half the time the molecules end up heads (cis) and half the time tails (trans), whereas within the plant, the chance of heads (cis) coming up is 100 percent. Slight variations of cis/trans ratios occur both on a random basis and in association with the total stereochemical structure of the fats. As a whole, heat extraction and hydrogenation result in random molecular changes of fats. Whenever vegetable- or seed-based fats are solid at room temperature, they have been hydrogenated, and so logically can be assumed to contain trans fatty acids. There are now products on the market that claim hydrogenation with fewer or no trans fatty acids. I am uncertain of the technology and remain skeptical that polyunsaturated oils can be safely hydrogenated.

It is not important that you understand the molecular chemistry of fats to appreciate the importance of these relationships. Trans fatty acids have been strongly linked to heart disease and cancer in both human and animal models. There is strong reason to believe that these are not the only diseases associated with inadequate essential fats and the intake of trans fatty acids. Many modern neuro-degenerative diseases, including Alzheimer's and multiple sclerosis, involve tissues with high fat content and a clear dependence on essential fats. It may someday be proved that the observed elevation of aluminum found in the brains of most Alzheimer's patients, yet not considered a cause of disease, is compounded and impactful when aluminum is bound to trans fatty acids in the frying pan and shows up in tissues as a more difficult toxin to eliminate. Many of your normal physiologic functions, including immunity and fertility, are dependent upon essential fats in the diet. Trans fatty acids have been shown to be incapable of serving in an essential manner and also to interfere with many normal physiologic processes.

To understand the logic of our scientific understanding of cis fatty acids, we only have to look at the structure of very important human chemicals like estrogen, progesterone, and testosterone. Like many other human chemicals, these hormones utilize a six-carbon ring wherein double-bonded carbons bend back upon each other until they reunite between the sixth and first carbon. Creation of this six-carbon ring structure of life is an impossibility with the trans fatty acid forms of fats found in the modern diet. Human studies have shown that it takes longer and utilizes more energy for the human body to process trans fatty acids out of the bloodstream and out of fat reserves. A graphic example of this chemical rigidity can be witnessed when you cook with polyunsaturated oils such as corn, safflower, canola, or flax oil The splattered oil from the frying pan is a firm resinous structure that requires much effort to remove from your appliances, unlike monosaturated oils such as olive oil that remain soft at higher temperatures. You should never cook essential fats at the higher temperatures required for frying, as you will then be producing your own trans fatty acids in your own kitchen. Trans fatty acids in the human diet have been strongly linked to a wide variety of degenerative diseases, yet we are still being told by oil companies and other organizations to use these polyunsaturated fats for cooking.

Different fats have different heat tolerances. I cannot list all food-grade oils and their appropriate extraction and cooking temperatures. A safe rule of thumb is to cook with olive oil and use cold-pressed vegetable and seed oils only in uncooked forms. Animal fats such as lard and bacon grease, although having their own downside, are in general more heat stable and therefore less harmful than cooking with polyunsaturated oils.

An increase in the essential fats can be gained by increasing your consumption of raw or lightly cooked vegetables. You can increase them even more by adding raw seeds like sunflower seeds to your basic diet, or you can guarantee an ample amount of these fats by supplementing your diet with cold-pressed seed oils like flax, sunflower, and borage. It is estimated that we need about 5 percent of our total daily calories in the form of essential fats. In a society that consumes 30–40 percent of our calories in fat, the average American does not get the 5 percent essential fat requirement. You may take care to reduce the "bad fats," but Americans are only recently understanding the importance of the essential oils of raw seeds and vegetables.

In the long run, I believe that medical science will clearly prove that the low-cost, heat-extracted vegetable and seed oils of modern times are far more harmful than animal fat. There are many sound reasons to decrease total as well as cholesterol-based fats in your diet, but the most important rule of thumb for fat intake is to provide adequate essential fats and minimal trans fatty acids in your diet.

Essential Amino Acids

Proteins are chemicals that contain one or more nitrogen atoms in their molecular structure. Daily protein needs include a group of essential amino acids, meaning that it is essential that humans consume these specific proteins as part of a normal diet. We cannot manufacture these specific amino acids or cannot manufacture adequate amounts of these proteins to maintain normal health, and therefore we must consume them as part of a total diet. There are eight essential amino acids for adults and nine that are recognized as essential to children. They are valine, lysine, threonine, leucine, isoleucine, tryptophan, phenylalanine, and methionine. Histidine is the amino acid required by infants, and some theorize it is also essential for adults. Most Americans get abundant if not excessive protein in their daily diet and specific deficiencies of essential amino acids are uncommon.

I mention essential amino acids for one reason. Years ago it was theorized that you needed to consume all eight essential amino acids at each given meal. This misconception followed the logical observation of ethnic diets that were unvaried, as in the Mexican staples of beans, rice, and corn. In combination, these three foods provide all eight essential amino acids in a healthy balance. Diets that don't vary and are based on a few foods that don't contain all eight essential proteins can lead to deficiencies of essential amino acids and therefore diseases of single protein deficiency. It is not necessary to consume all eight at every meal to maintain health. If you eat corn on Monday, brown rice on Tuesday, and beans on Wednesday, your body will do just fine. Eating a variety of whole foods with adequate total protein is a much easier approach than trying to chart out all eight amino acids for each meal.

Lecithin

Though not typically listed with essential micronutrients, lecithin is an important nutrient that is found abundantly in egg yolks and legumes (beans like soy, pinto, aduki, black, and kidney). Lecithin is an important component of cell walls, nerve cells, and digestive function. You don't need to supplement this food if you have an abundance of legumes in your daily diet.

Vitamins, Minerals, and Enzymes

Vitamins and minerals have long been recognized as essential nutrients for humans. There continues to be great debate about what represents the optimum level of intake for vitamins. A general consensus exists that the current U.S. RDAs, or recommended daily allowances, are low for many of the common vitamins. The RDAs for minerals are generally considered to be not only adequate, but within optimal levels as well. Certain trace minerals like selenium, zinc, and chromium are gaining added support for their roles in preventing many diseases. The role of live enzymes, particularly those found in fresh vegetables, is also gaining broad support within the general public, although these important nutrients are lagging far behind both vitamins and minerals as generally accepted required nutrients.

Vitamins are divided into two categories. Fat-soluble vitamins include vitamins A, D, E, and K with all other vitamins being water-soluble. With the fat-soluble vitamins, there exists a potential for harm from excessive intake. This is primarily associated with vitamin A, as this vitamin is a fat-soluble molecule that can only be stored in the liver. Intake resulting in excessive levels of stored vitamin A can result in liver damage or death. Though rare, great caution should be taken in exceeding the RDA of vitamin A. Vitamin D is often called a provitamin, because humans can manufacture this molecule with adequate exposure to sunlight. It may be an important contributor to adequate maintenance of bone density, as well as performing other important regulatory actions. Only vitamin E among the fat-soluble vitamins has an RDA that is clearly too low for optimum health. While it does have the potential to elevate blood pressure in high doses, most nutritionists recommend a daily intake of 200–400 international units (IUs).

This book is not about the complete understanding of vitamins, and I only provide a brief overview. For more detailed information, consistent with the goals of optimal nutrition, I recommend the following resources:

- *Diet and Nutrition, a Holistic Approach.* Rudolph Ballentine, M.D. Himalayan Press.
- *Nutrition Against Disease: Environmental Protection.* Roger John Williams, M.D. Bantam.
- *Staying Healthy with Nutrition: The Complete Guide to Diet and Nutritional Medicine.* Elson Haas, M.D. Celestial Arts.
- *The Nutrition Almanac.* Gayla Kirschmann and John Kirschmann. McGraw-Hill.
- *Modern Nutrition in Health and Disease.* Maurice E. Shills, M.D., Editor. Lippincott, Williams & Wilkins.

The water-soluble vitamins include all other vitamins, including the Bs (B_1 or thiamine, B_2 or riboflavin, B_3 or niacin, B_6 or pyridoxine, and B_{12}), beta-carotene, pantothenic acid, folic acid, and vitamin C. This is the area where most people question the adequacy of the RDA standards. Contemporary authors suggest that the RDA of most B vitamins is about one-tenth the optimal level and that the RDA of vitamin C may be one-hundredth of the optimal daily allowance. You can provide higher levels of these vitamins by the intake of more nutritious foods, but it is difficult with a modern diet to match the levels achieved by our ancestors. Supplementation is not only logical but is critical insurance for good long-term health.

Webster's defines enzyme as "any of various organic substances that are produced in plant and animal cells and cause changes in other substances by catalytic action."[2] Enzymes as components of our diet have been recognized as important in the prevention of disease since the 1940s. At that time, Dr. William Pottinger, a medical researcher, showed that fresh vegetables, when added to the diet of his laboratory animals, significantly reduced their long-term incidences of cancer, cardiovascular disease, and a number of conditions we label as Western diseases. In spite of the quality of his research and the importance of his discoveries, this area of required nutrition has only recently emerged in mainstream consciousness. Without question, one of the richest sources of live enzymes can be found in fresh vegetable juices.

Biologics

Though it is not considered a standard classification of nutrition, the term *biologics* refers to the beneficial bacteria and yeasts of our ancestral diet. These bacteria and their benefits are discussed in greater detail in Chapter 2, but they are worth a second mention. Nearly every human culture has a history of fermented or cultured products that are an important part of their diet. As discussed in *The Bacillus of Long Life*, Douglas, 1911, the bacteria and yeasts of these products often vary with the cultures, but in all cases they present a wide array of friendly microbes that aid digestion and help to prevent various infections and diseases. Many of these products have involved fermented or cultured milk products, including yogurt, but they also include the cultured cabbage of Asian and European heritage as well as fermented beans and other food sources. By continually reseeding friendly microbes in our bodies, we are helping to offset the current rampage of antibiotics and steroids in the Western diet.

Herbs and Edible Fungi

While there are herbal and fungal products and extracts that have true medicinal actions, most herbs and fungi deserve to be given nutritional appreciation. There is little difference between most herbs and fungi and other foods we eat. Eating garlic, for example, can help with cholesterol levels and decrease undesired yeast growth, and garlic adds a unique flavor to foods as well. Many of the culinary seasonings that we call "spices" aid digestion by increasing the overall flavor of a meal and therein stimulating more active secretion of digestive enzymes. In addition, some herbal products provide phytosterols, which assist your own hormonal balance. Many of the therapeutic actions of plants that we experience may simply be compensation for their chronic absence from today's daily diet. In seeking variety, remember mushrooms and herbs as our ancestors did.

Nutrition and Disease

There are very few diseases that are not influenced by nutrition. Not only does nutrition play a key role in how well you deal with life's stresses, but also many conditions show clear benefits from improved eating habits and the use of supplemental nutrients. Modern research does a great disservice to the power of nutrition by using a reductionistic model of investigation. There are so many interactions between essential nutrients and normal function that research into single-nutrient relationships and chronic disease is blatantly limited in its ability to review and define complete nutritional impact on disease. While single-nutrient disease states will continue to be revealed by this method of inquiry, the complex interactions of all the important nutrients will always evade this model.

While there is ample scientific evidence of the role of nutrition in disease, there remains a wide variety of views on the complete importance of these relationships. Some people minimize both the severity of impact from poor nutrition as well as the efficacy and importance of nutritional changes. Everyone agrees that certain levels of vitamins and minerals are required for health but again there exists much disagreement on the levels needed and whether therapeutic nutrition can be accomplished through diet alone. I believe that supplemental nutrition is not only logical but also essential in this day and age. While understanding the presence of biochemical individuality and the lack of consensus on optimal levels of micronutrients, I have generally used the following supplemental approach for my patients.

Daily Power Blend

1 medium-sized whole fruit (apple, banana, etc.)
½ to 1 cup fruit juice or appropriate liquid (use 100 percent juice, rice milk, soy milk, etc.)
1 to 2 tablespoons yogurt

In a blender, combine all the ingredients.

This is a carrying vehicle for the added supplements listed below. The purpose is to provide a pleasant-tasting smoothie that can be appreciated on a regular basis.

To the smoothie, add:

1 tablespoon cold-pressed flaxseed oil
1 heaping teaspoon lecithin granules
1 tablespoon protein powder
2 to 4 capsules Nutrizyme™
7 drops liquid beta-carotene

I developed this combination about fifteen years ago after observing many of my cancer and AIDS patients swallowing handfuls of tablets and capsules every day to supplement their diet with the hopes of helping their disease condition. I remembered that the M.D. who taught me diagnosis and minor surgery in naturopathic medical school had shared a personal story in one of these classes. He told us that a man he hired to clean his septic tank reported that it was common to find one to two inches of prescription and nonprescription tablets and capsules at the bottom of septic tanks. Truly, what you put in your mouth doesn't always end up in your body. Knowing that my AIDS and cancer patients often had more problems than most with general digestion, I felt it was essential to eliminate this significant variable from supplemental therapy. I chose to ensure the most basic nutritional needs in an easily absorbed, liquid form.

I have found that most people rapidly experience a personal increase in energy and overall health when they drink this smoothie on a regular basis. If nutrition is considered in economic terms, this combination not only provides the day's expenses but also simultaneously retires nutritional debt and begins investment into nutritional reserves. From a micronutrient basis this drink provides the nutrition of about six normal meals, with the calories of one, and the digestive effort of about one-third of that required for a normal meal. It's like getting a holiday bonus every day of the year. I recommend this drink five days a week for therapeutic purposes and three days a week for health maintenance. I have one AIDS patient who has improved steadily for the past seven years, using this drink seven days a week, twice daily. It does not contain nutrients that would provide toxic effects at higher frequency, so feel free to use it daily or even more if you desire. I use five days a week as a normal recommendation, so people can still go out to occasional breakfasts with friends and also so people don't burn out on a rigid routine.

The flaxseed oil is an excellent source of essential fats while the lecithin and protein powder combine with the essential fats and existing cholesterol to provide readily available nutrients for the repair and production of healthy cell walls and other important structures. These four things provide close to 95 percent of the chemicals found in our cell wall membranes. With improvements in essential fats and lecithin, the membranes are purported to be less sensitive to oxidative and chemical damage as well as more fluid in the transport of nutrients and wastes across the membrane.

Nutrizyme, from Tyler Encapsulations, is a professional supplement, available across the United States and Canada, that not only provides an excellent balance of vitamins and minerals but also supplies live vegetable enzymes. While these enzymes have been shown to be important in maintaining health and preventing the incidence of many diseases, they also aid the digestion and absorption of this blend, so that even people with impaired digestion show improved absorption.

I have found in clinical practice that the liquid form of beta-carotene is either more absorbable or more biologically active than tablets or capsules commonly available at nutrition outlets. Beta-carotene when converted to vitamin A is a major player in DNA transcription, and thus in the production of new cells. Natural beta-carotene has never been linked to vitamin A toxicity, and has a wide range of safe levels of intake. When you reach the serum level where you show an orange coloring, it is the reflection of light off this orange molecule and is not related to the yellow jaundice of hepatitis, including vitamin A–induced liver damage. If you reach the orange level you have more than enough beta-carotene in your system and reduction in the level of intake is a logical step.

Finally, I recommend that people not start with a soy-based protein powder. Even before the emergence of the high level of GMO soy in the American market, I have found whole soybeans and soy powder to be a very difficult protein for many people to digest. Frequently when a person uses the soy-base product on a long-term basis, his or her body begins to struggle with the relationship. Sometimes a queasy feeling, sometimes nausea, and occasionally flu-like symptoms will develop with long-term use. While soy is an excellent food as a whole, the soymilk and tofu forms seem more easily handled by the average person. I have recommended that my patients use a product sold in the United States by a company named Naturade and marketed as soy-free vegetable protein. Once the power blend has been successfully introduced, I leave it to the individual patient to consider use of soy, egg-based powders, or other protein-powder combination. I have no economic interest or involvement with Tyler Encapsulations or Naturade.

As additional supplementation to the power blend, I recommend 200–400 IUs vitamin E, 1,000–2,000 mg vitamin C, and 500 mg calcium/ 250 mg magnesium. For postmenopausal women, 1,000 mg calcium/500 mg magnesium.

Long-Term Goals and Daily Habits

For most people, energy and an absence of disease are their overall health goals. To accomplish these goals in the simplest, or least laborious, manner is the preferred approach. We like to enjoy our day-to-day lives, and most people don't want to spend a lot of time and energy counting calories, planning meals from a rigid standard of nutrition, or eating foods that don't appeal to them. It is important that you have a dietary approach that fits your lifestyle, your time constraints, and your budget. Most people want to enjoy their meals and feel energized by their consumption.

In the twenty-plus years that I have helped people with their diet, I have found that starting with the familiar is the most effective route to long-term success. Instead of providing an ideal daily meal plan, I start with having patients record a one-week diet diary and from this information, suggest a few beneficial changes. These are typically similar suggestions of increasing water and fluids, increasing the amounts of crunchy vegetables, and broadening the variety of cereals, grains, and seeds. Taking small steps, recognizing the benefits, and continuing the journey results in great long-term improvements and doesn't leave you lost in the unfamiliar. Too many people try to take giant steps and fail to realize their long-term objectives.

There are many clinical indicators of proper nutrition. These include weight, serum cholesterol, cholesterol ratios, homocysteine levels, and red blood cell counts along with an array of metabolic enzymes and organ function tests. These are important indices, but your own subjective awareness of energy, creativity, mental clarity, and wellness are invaluable aids to assuring ideal nutrition. If you have never experienced an ideal state of health, it is hard to evaluate how close you are to your best diet. Hopefully, the fasting diet will begin to give you a more complete measuring stick for how good you can feel.

Whenever the subject of organic foods is introduced, the topic of expense arises. My favorite response is that the true cost of organic produce is found at the checkout counter, whereas the cost of nonorganic foods is continued over time with poor health, disease, and decreased life productivity. I have never found a patient with serious health concerns or severe disease that has found money saved to be a replacement for his or her lost health. The "penny wise, pound foolish" quote of Benjamin Franklin is no more apropos than when it is applied to diet and lifestyle.

In his 1903 book *Return to Nature*, Adolf Just writes about the natural diet and what he and other early naturopaths referred to as "nature cure." He contends, like many early naturopaths, that the human system is not suited to consume beef and other animal products. Writing that the smell of a ripe strawberry will please and stimulate most people's appetites, he notes that standing next to and smelling a cow never stimulates an enhanced appetite response. He adds that we have to cook the animal in tasty spices and salt to make it appealing and that unseasoned meats are rarely attractive to those who haven't already developed a taste for prepared flesh.

Lyndon Smith, M.D., famous pediatrician and author, has maintained for years that the senses of smell and taste are invaluable indicators of nutritional need. He incorporated this belief into practice by having his patients smell individual vitamins and nutrients to establish their optimal supplemental balance. While poor nutrition can produce an unhealthy taste for refined sugar, salt, or other foods, when we have taken a few steps to a better diet, these cravings or desires are often changed into a more appropriate relationship with foods. Other writers have suggested that the state of energy immediately following a meal is a strong indicator of its true worth to the system. Nutrition is not rocket science and the use of common sense, basic knowledge, and an awareness of your response to foods is often the only road map you need for a successful journey to improved health.

Your own life journey is defined by the choices you make. Like trails on the path of life, you try to make choices that are consistent with your own desired destination. You integrate your values, experience, and knowledge and do your best to choose trails that don't lead you far astray. When you find yourself in the brambles (disease, fatigue, dependency, or addiction), you backtrack and set off again. In awareness of mistakes comes the knowledge of the experienced guide.

How you choose to live goes far beyond your own physical experience. Your health impacts how well you live and support your family and community; it impacts how soon and to what degree your children and grandchildren go from dependents to caregivers; and it impacts the planet we live on. If you choose a conscious simplification of your diet, you not only feel better physically, but emotionally as well.

The Hygienists, nature curists, and early naturopaths generally advocated a whole foods diet with few or no animal products. Milk and fermented dairy were the primary animal products recommended by those who did advocate a nonvegetarian diet. The milk was of course organic and was not yet pasteurized. All animals were what we now call "free range," which is an important consideration if you do choose to include meat in your diet. Free range refers to animals that are raised in open versus penned environments. With exercise and a more varied diet, these animals are generally less in need of antibiotics and steroids. As animals, like humans, tend to store and accumulate these chemicals in their tissues, you can significantly reduce your exposure to these chemicals by eating less commercially produced dairy and meats.

Mindful of world hunger we try to solve this problem from a global economic and political perspective. While decade after decade, feeding animals enough to feed the planet, while using enough grain in the production of alcohol to feed the planet, we fail to feed the men, women, and children of all nations. A well-nourished society is a safer and healthier society for us all.

Reversal of disease may require a specialized approach to diet, but to maintain good health most of us can serve as our own nutritionist. Considering the proven biochemical individuality of humans, the relationship of taste and smell to optimal digestive and immune function, possible genetic variables, as suggested in *Eat Right 4 Your Type* by Dr. D'Adamo or even the body-type diets of the Ayurvedic system, you are ultimately the best judge of your relationship with any given food. With these varied unknowns, the basic four, mentioned at the beginning of this chapter, can serve you well in your long, easy journey to optimum health.

- Whole and organic foods are the best.
- Variety is very important.
- Minimize the processing and cooking of your foods.
- Pay attention to your individual response to foods.

Good Shopping Habits

A key to establishing a healthy diet is to develop good shopping habits. Think ahead: how often will you eat on the run or snack between meals?

How often will you need to prepare a quick meal for the family? What are your favorite healthy meals? Choosing wholesome snacks, having a good selection of staples, and an abundance of fruits and vegetables makes meal planning much simpler.

By whole foods, I mean unprocessed whole grains and cereals, and foods as they present in nature, not in the can, freezer case, or additive-saturated prepared products. In the whole and organic form, foods are most likely to carry the complete nutrition that we can thrive upon. They are also less likely to contribute to pesticide-linked cancers and disease and are much less likely to include the unproven GMOs.

Label reading is an essential skill of modern times. Unfortunately, label reading is not always the end of the story. Years ago my wife brought a loaf of bread home from a vacation trip. The bread was marked "no artificial preservatives." It sat, unattended, at room temperature for over a month. Upon reopening it was still soft, mold-free, and obviously well preserved. It was then that I discovered that if a baker called a chemical a "dough freshener," a "flavor enhancer," or any other acceptable term, he could label his product as free of artificial preservatives. Bread should get stale and or moldy if left for days in open air. If it stays soft and fresh for weeks, there are added chemicals.

We have some very good laws and regulations governing the production and preparation of food, but they are by no means perfect. When it comes to chemical additives, the United States is one of the most lenient nations in the Western world. While we recognize that these chemicals can inhibit the oxidative actions of molds and bacterial oxidation, their proof of safety lies in limited human and animal exposure to single chemicals, with a short-term evaluation of toxicity and allergic response. There is not a required evaluation standard that looks at the multi-chemical interactions of these additives in the "real world"— human diet. While we recognize that these chemicals impair microbial oxidation (spoilage), we don't ask how they might influence the necessary enzymatic oxidation of digestion. It is again your choice of whether you believe these chemicals to be safe, or of an undetermined safety. Your vote is cast and counted at the checkout stand.

Variety, as the spice of life, is also the essence of health. Try new foods, include edible mushrooms and fungi and as many different vegetables, fruits, cereals, grains, and seeds as your resources allow. We may never know or isolate the many different important nutrients found in the different species of plants or fungi. Fungi have shown important nutrients, called beta-glucans, that have proven to be potent immune stimulators, as well as quality protein and fiber.

Processing, including cooking, is generally associated with a reduction of nutritional content. Some foods like beans, mushrooms, winter squash, and many others require some degree of cooking to make the nutrients digestible and usable by humans. It is important to not overcook these foods and find that middle ground where the nutrients are usable, but not destroyed.

Do You Like It?

Your own response to foods not only includes your subjective responses from a physical perspective, but also includes whether they satisfy your appetite and tastes. We need pleasurable feedback to maintain a long-term relationship with a given food.

8

Helpful Additions to Your Fast

This book outlines the foundations for fasting, and I recommend that they be strictly observed. After completing the pre-fast diet, which requires a lot of food preparation, you enter into the juice phase, which is much easier and less time consuming. Typically while on juices, you will experience an increase in energy while requiring less sleep and less time for food preparation, eating, and overall kitchen cleanup. This additional time, coupled with the calm energy of a fast, is an excellent time to explore physical, spiritual, and emotional practices that can improve your fasting and detoxing experience.

There are many pleasurable and beneficial activities that you can safely add to your power-fast program. When leading the extended Passage 23 program, I have offered morning yoga classes and provided participants with one massage, one colonic, and one skin care treatment. I also encourage participants to explore other avenues of support and nurturing during their fasts. Some of the common adjuncts are discussed in this chapter.

Massage

Today's consumer often overlooks massage, one of the oldest forms of traditional medicine. The reasons for this oversight are the relative lack of medical and public exposure given to this practice, and the inappropriate fear that massage is a sexual practice. Limited insurance coverage for preventive care like massage results in consumers having to pay for therapy themselves. This financial disincentive also works against massage gaining its rightful place in current medicine.

Massage has a rich history in virtually all cultures. It evolved side-by-side with acupuncture and other eastern systems. In Western medicine, references to massage date back to Homer in 1200 B.C. and Hippocrates in 460 B.C. American authors and practitioners like Dr. J. H. Kellogg wrote entire books on massage and advocated its use as an important component of health care.

The *Manual of Hydrotherapy and Massage*, by Dr. Fred Moor, defines massage as "the manipulation of the tissues of the body for therapeutic purposes." The beneficial effects of massage include improved circulation, improved lymphatic drainage (waste removal, immune support), muscle relaxation, and stress reduction. Human skin-to-skin contact, as in massage, has been shown to release endorphins, which elevate both mood and immune function. Reduction of stress, in and of itself, offers many health benefits associated with the cardiovascular system, the musculoskeletal system, and the immune system. Some studies have cited increased immune function from massage as well as an increase in the production of beneficial and pleasurable endorphins.

The most common type of massage practiced in America is called Swedish massage. It utilizes a number of strokes that generally increase circulation and lymph drainage and counteract muscle tension. Other types of massage are used singularly or in conjunction with Swedish techniques. Shiatsu is a Japanese pressure-point technique similar to acupressure, the Chinese system that uses pressure on particular points to improve the electrical and energy systems of the body. Polarity therapy is an Indian system of energy massage, while Trager technique utilizes gentle rocking and range of motion to help release emotional tensions. Rolfing is a very deep muscle pressure technique, which involves pressure to trigger points of the muscles, leading to relaxation and ultimately the rebalancing of posture. There are numerous other forms of massage with long and effective histories of practice.

Even within a particular massage practice, there exist differences between individual practitioners. Most states have licensure and practice laws regulating the field of massage. This is an important standard of competency, but it does not guarantee the skill level of a given practitioner. While you may find some practitioners or types of massage that don't appeal to you, hopefully you will find those that do provide benefit. With all types of massage therapy, you should expect a clean environment and a professional regard for your privacy and modesty (gowns and appropriate draping). Therapists often use oil to decrease friction between their hands and your skin. If you have sensitivities to particular oils or fragrances make certain to mention this before your massage.

Getting a massage during a fast is an excellent idea. Not only are you typically more limber and therefore less tender to deep work, but you have an excellent opening to your intuition and spirit. You can often make breakthroughs in emotional holding patterns while using the benefits of lymphatic drainage and detoxification, which are stimulated by many forms of massage. It is also a great time for energy massage like shiatsu, acupressure, polarity, or Reiki techniques.

Hydrotherapy

Hydrotherapy is simply the use of water for therapeutic benefits. It includes the more common therapies like hot tubs, Jacuzzis, steam rooms, and saunas. It also includes the wet-sheet wrap and combination therapies of hot and cold applications as well as the use of microcurrent in conjunction with the heat and cold.

The basic principle of hydrotherapy is to use temperature to improve circulation to aid in repair and detoxification. There are many spas and facilities that provide sophisticated programs, but you can gain benefit from the equipment most people have at home. Sitz baths, hot baths with Epson salts, or hot baths followed by a cold shower are a few of the hydrotherapies available at no or little cost.

The number of books on the many different types of hydrotherapy programs that exist will surprise you. I leave it to you to further your knowledge of these therapies and to choose the ones that work best for you. In general, when fasting, you have a slightly lower tolerance for heat. If you do not commonly use hot tubs or saunas, use caution not to exceed your heat tolerance. Work your way up to longer and hotter, and use a conservative common sense when initiating these practices. It is not necessary to use the hottest temperatures to assist detoxification; lower temperatures, like the lower bench of most saunas, maintained for a longer period of time may actually be more effective. The sebaceous glands of the skin, not the sweat glands, release the most toxins. The term "sweating out toxins" is somewhat of a misnomer, in that the sweat glands serve to diffuse heat and to protect your brain from too high of a core body temperature. Lower temperatures maintained for a longer period of time are the best environments for sebaceous gland elimination.

Yoga

Yoga literally means "union" and is an Eastern practice of unifying the body, breath, and mind with the Creator. There are many Eastern practices that combine movement, breathing, and mental discipline within a spiritual system. Chi Gong and Tai Chi are two of the popular methods being practiced in current times. Like aerobic exercise, you may find some practices that "feel" right and others that don't. It is very hard to practice a form of yoga or other meditative discipline on a long-term basis if it doesn't fit with your personal needs. Investigate what is out there until you find one or more that truly work for you.

I began practicing yoga in 1968. I didn't know I was doing yoga at the time and neither did the other young men on my wrestling team. We just knew that we were doing the stretches that our coach told us had helped keep his teams from frequent injuries over the years. Our teams had fewer injuries (we were always able to field two healthy wrestlers at all weight classifications) and I maintain that the conditioning and stretching were significant contributions to our team's physical health.

In 1972 I took my first formal class in hatha yoga. I immediately recognized the positions, or asanas, as being identical to many of the stretches from our wrestling practices. In yoga, there are not only common positions for each exercise, but also specific breathing for each positional change. These practices long predate my wrestling experiences and the breathing techniques are orthopedically sound and purposeful. It is valuable to find a skilled yoga instructor to refine the simple breathing of your practice. We are most familiar with the discipline of hatha yoga, as it has been the most common yoga practice of public television and college courses. There are many different types of yoga practice, some of which only involve breathing techniques, and not stretches or specific asanas.

I have found pleasure and benefit from many different types of yoga. Yoga can have a spiritual base, and many of the disciplines do come with a spiritual side, but the breathing and passive stretching of yoga is beneficial from a strictly physical standpoint. You will find that during a fast you have much greater flexibility and that yoga is an easier practice than at nonfasting times.

One of my favorite yoga stretches is the "sun worship," which is outlined below. I have also included a few specific purification and elimination exercises from tantric yoga. You may wish to read up on yoga or find your local yoga society and connect with a personal instructor.

Other resources include:

3HO Foundation
International Headquarters
House of Guru Ram Das
1620 Preuss Road
Los Angeles, CA 90035

Kundalini Research Institute
c/o G.T. International
1800 South Robertson Boulevard, Suite 182
Los Angeles, CA 90035
(213) 551-0484

SRF
Self-Realization Fellowship
3880 San Raphael Avenue
Los Angeles, CA 90065

The Sun Worship

The sun worship is a smooth movement through many extensions and flexions of the whole body. It employs a very simple breath technique and is neither complicated, nor extreme in its positional requirements. As its name would imply, it is an excellent starting stretch for any yoga or daily routine.

Position One is simply standing comfortably with palms of hands joined in front of your sternum or heart. (See Figure 8.1.) While in this position take an initial few deep, relaxed breaths trying to expand both inhalation and exhalation volumes—almost as much inhalation as you would take to hold your breath and almost as much exhalation as if you were slowly blowing out all the candles on a birthday cake. The breath

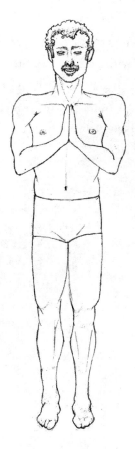
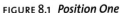

FIGURE 8.1 *Position One*

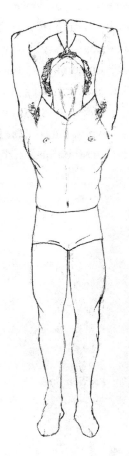

FIGURE 8.2 *Position Two*

should be smooth in its transition from inhalation to exhalation and back. It is not a rapid breath that could lead to hyperventilation. As you complete the exhalation, you are ready to inhale as you move into Position Two (Figure 8.2).

As you reach your full comfortable extension, you should be reaching completion of a full inhalation. The full breath is an important structural support for the spinal pressure of extension. Extension positions throughout this exercise are always accompanied by inspiration. With a fluid movement, you leave this position as you begin to exhale, moving into Position Three (Figure 8.3).

As your hands and body move toward your toes, you are completely emptying your lungs so that you can bend with greater flexibility. Your breath should be empty, and inhalation begins as you lift one foot to extend your leg behind you while placing both palms to the floor for support as shown in Figure 8.4. Position Four is again a spinal extension and should be accompanied with a full inhalation.

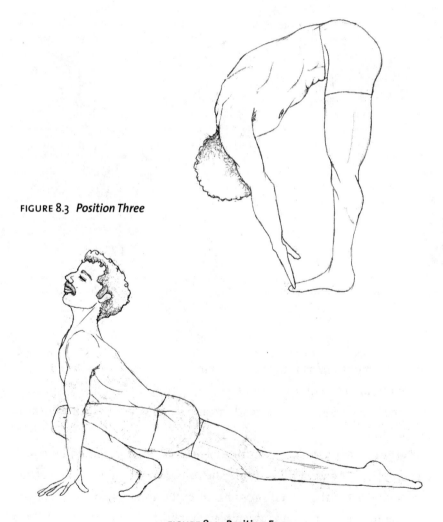

FIGURE 8.3 *Position Three*

FIGURE 8.4 *Position Four*

The amount of extension in this position is that which can be accomplished without pain and without outside force or momentum. Yoga is not a contest; it is a union of your own breath and body and is expanded with practice, not force. From Position Four, you simultaneously begin exhalation as you bring the bent leg back with the straightened leg and continue into Position Five, which is a very relaxed forward flexion (Figure 8.5).

Position Five moves into the most strenuous extension of the series, Position Six (Figure 8.6). People with low back problems should adjust

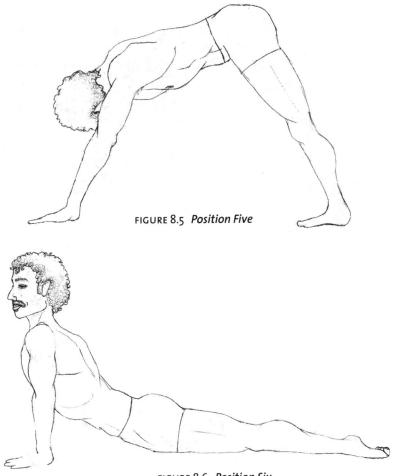

FIGURE 8.5 *Position Five*

FIGURE 8.6 *Position Six*

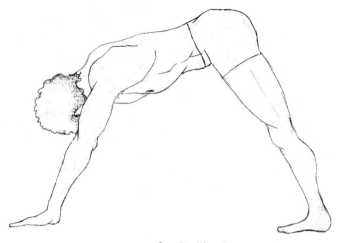

FIGURE 8.7 *Position Seven*

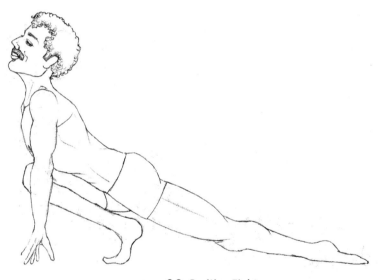

FIGURE 8.8 *Position Eight*

this stretch so that they are on their knees to establish a less forceful pressure on their lumbar vertebrae. Again, it is essential that you have a full breath when you enter into this extension.

As you begin to exhale in Position Six you return to the easy flexion of Position Five (Figure 8.7), reaching full flexion with the complete exhalation.

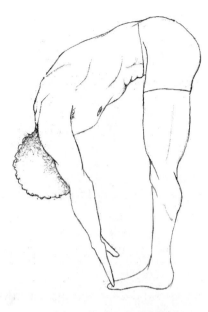

FIGURE 8.9 *Position Nine*

From Position Seven you begin an inhalation as you move into Position Eight (Figure 8.8). Position Eight is identical to Position Four, except the opposite leg is brought forward to achieve a balanced stretch of both right and left legs and pelvis. I've never read or heard that there is any importance to whether the right leg or the left leg goes back first in this series. Position Four starts with the left leg back, but could easily start with the right leg back. The important thing is to reverse order between Positions Four and Eight.

From Position Eight, you return with exhalation to the toe touching posture of Position Three (Figure 8.9).

As you complete the sequence with a final inhalation, you return to the original starting position (Position One) and breath. You can repeat this series as many times as you like. You will often notice greater flexibility as you repeat the sequence and you will notice greater flexibility throughout your day. You are using your breath with your body and mind to set the foundation for a great day.

The sun worship is commonly taught in hatha yoga but is widely utilized by a number of disciplines. The following asanas are more specialized techniques for your fasting experience. They are techniques I have learned through practice and study. Many of them are from the Kundalini and Tantric disciplines and most are covered with greater content in the excellent practice guide *Sadhana Guidelines for Kundalini Yoga Daily Practice*, Arcline Publications.

Abdominal and Eliminatory Support

The next two movements are especially helpful for digestive activity and abdominal lymph flow. The first, called the "cat cow" (Figure 8.10) is a simple exercise where you assume a position on your hands and knees. As you exhale, you move into the cat position, which is similar to the frightened cat images of Halloween, except that in yoga and in anatomy, the neck is part of the back. When you arch your back, you also bend your head and neck forward. As you inhale you move into the cow position with back and neck extending fully. Repeat with each full breath.

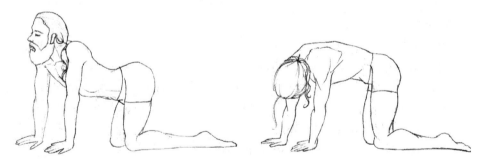

FIGURE 8.10 *Cat Cow*

The next exercise starts in a comfortable cross-legged position with your fingers touching your shoulders (Figure 8.11). Inhale through the nose and twist to the left; exhale out the mouth and twist to the right. You are once again using a relaxed deep breath. Twist from your waist,

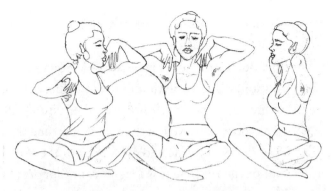

FIGURE 8.11 *Abdominal Twist*

allowing the momentum of your shoulders to rotate your torso, stretching across your back. This rapid inhalation-exhalation accompanied by the release of back tension is wonderfully energizing and helps support abdominal function, lymph drainage, and overall detoxification.

Purification Exercises

The last three techniques that I'm providing in this very limited section on yoga are purification, or cleansing and balancing, positions. They are primarily stationary exercises with the breath being the primary focus. I have had various teachers use different breathing techniques for all three asanas, and you may safely choose any of the following patterns.

The first and easiest technique is the same deep relaxed breath of the previous exercises. Another common breath that is more powerful in its action is a faster, more exaggerated breath in which you inhale as you pull your abdomen in and up and exhale as you push your abdomen out. Often this technique will be accompanied by the Sat Nam chant of yogic practice. One last technique involves a slow, metered breath where you inhale in sixteen equal steps and exhale in sixteen equal breaths. This really helps in controlling your breathing and often assists other techniques. Often my students will start with twelve breaths of inhalation and exhalation and work up to sixteen.

The first purification technique (Figure 8.12) is practiced in a comfortable sitting position. Placing the thumb over one nostril you inhale fully. Release the thumb from the nostril and place the "pinky" finger over the opposite nostril as you exhale. Repeat this many times and then change hands and nostrils so that you inhale and exhale out of the opposite nostrils. Increasing your oxygen exchange is a significant support to the benefits of fasting. It aids in elimination, acid-base balance, and in overall energy delivery to all your cells and their functional demands.

Another easy purification exercise is shown in Figure 8.13. In a comfortable kneeling position you interlace your hands as shown, raising them high above your head while maintaining good spinal position. You can use any of the aforementioned breathing techniques as you sustain this single position.

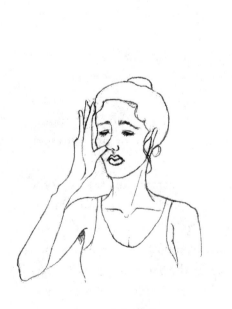

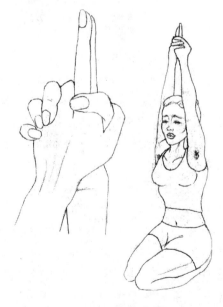

FIGURE 8.12

First Purification Position

FIGURE 8.13

Second Purification Position

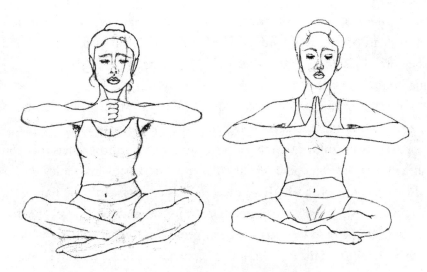

FIGURE 8.14 *Breathing Position*

The final exercise, shown in Figure 8.14, involves two different sustained positions and is best practiced with either the deep relaxed breath or the metered sixteen-interval breath. In the first position, you are sitting comfortably as you grasp your fingers together while pulling them apart. The traction is to be maintained throughout your many breaths with steady strength and unmoving position. The balancing follow-up to this position involves placing your palms together as you push them together with ongoing breaths. Again the pressure and position should be maintained throughout the cycles of breath.

Exercise

It is safe and pleasant to exercise while on the fasting diet. As a working-class fast, it not only provides you the energy for normal work requirements, but for exercise as well. Many of my fasting participants have been avid runners or competitive in other sports. One college varsity runner set her personal records for five thousand and ten thousand meters while on the juice phase of this program. She found that her training runs of more than twenty miles were difficult, but like most fasters, she found the normal distances to be easier and her rebound to be quicker than during nonfasting times.

It is important to begin exercising with moderation. If you currently are not accustomed to aerobic training, do not push yourself to exhaustion. A general rule of thumb for starting an exercise program is that you should feel like you could repeat an exercise activity within a few hours of ceasing your program. If you feel exhausted long after you have quit, you probably pushed yourself too hard. Back off and find a level of activity that can be built upon as a regular program. Keep it fun; if you don't like running, try dancing, swimming, or whatever feels good and is pleasurable enough to maintain on a regular basis.

Homeopathy

Homeopathy is a resurgent field of medicine, fast returning to the American medical system. Its name is descriptive of its philosophy, which is based on the principle of "like curing like," or what is called the "law of similars." *Homeo*, meaning same, and *pathy*, meaning disease, is the name given this field of medicine by its creator, Dr. Samuel Hahnemann. In 1790 Dr. Hahnemann was working on revising a *materia medica*, or materials of medicine, when he noticed that the toxic actions of an herb called china, *Cinchona officinalis*, were identical to the condition that it so effectively treated. China, or quinine, remains the major category or therapeutic treatment for malaria and is still used by orthodox medicine, called allopathy, to treat malaria. Dr. Hahnemann noticed that when people consumed toxic levels of china, they produced night sweats, intermittent fever, and had fatigue. These are the major symptoms of malaria, which can be controlled by therapeutic dosages of the same herb.

Dr. Hahnemann was intrigued and fascinated by this apparent paradox within medicine. He found that many of the commonly effective medicines of the time had a similar relationship between the symptoms of toxicity and the symptoms of the diseases that they effectively treated. He recognized that medicine used a lower, nontoxic dosage in the management of disease and wondered what would be the ideal dosage of medicine for the highest effectiveness of care. Before embarking on this issue he went through a rigorous testing of china on himself to make certain that the toxic presentations of this herb were in fact the symptoms listed in the various *materia medicas* of the time. As he consumed china over a number of days he did indeed begin to experience night sweats, intermittent fever, and fatigue. Over the next fifty years he experimented with ninety-nine drugs and recorded their actions on the human body. He published these findings in his book *Fragmenta de Viribus Medicamentorum Positivis*. Throughout his rigorous study and experimentation he became absolutely convinced of the "law of similars" as a guide to the ideal choice of medicines for the treatment of disease. The "law of similars" is of course a close cousin to the "Doctrine of Signatures," dating back to Hippocrates and earlier traditional medicines.

What distinguished this new approach to medicine was Hahnemann's understanding of effective dosage and the creation of the homeopathic principle called the "law of minimum dose." Hahnemann found that when a plant-, mineral-, or animal-based drug's action most closely matched the individual expression of disease, you could use less of the specific drug with better long-term results. He published these findings and theories in his famous book *Organon of Medicine*, which included six revised editions during his lifetime. The *Organon of Medicine* remains as the foundation of all current homeopathic practice. It also served as the source of criticism and later conversion by one Dr. Herring who in his attempt to discredit homeopathy became one of its most noted leaders. As Dr. Herring challenged the principles of homeopathy with sound scientific investigation, he found its safety and efficacy to be far better than the drug treatments of his time. He added the "law of cure" to the homeopathic paradigm and remains an important figure in the roots of this medicine.

There are many practitioners and resources for the study and practice of homeopathy. It is less regulated in the United States than in many countries so there may not be a certification process required in an individual state. Always feel free to ask any practitioner about his or her education or training regarding any therapy. Low-potency homeopathic medicines are available over-the-counter for first aid and minor health concerns, but the more potent, "constitutional" remedies require the services of a skilled homeopath.

Fasting is one of the greatest tools for the effective use of homeopathic medicines. Not only do you present with a clearer picture of your underlying health problems, but your body is much more responsive to the subtle yet powerful actions of homeopathic medicines. It is certainly not important that you include homeopathic medicines during a fast. You will still receive great benefit from the changes that occur from a successful fasting experience.

Acupuncture

Like homeopathy, the energy systems influenced by acupuncture are greatly eased during a fast and therefore much more responsive to treatment. A major fact to remember if considering this choice of medicine is that many acupuncturists do not advocate juice fasting. They often speak of the condition of a damp spleen, which is a common diagnosis in the Western world. The dietary recommendations for this condition exclude juices and the acupuncturist might cast doubts on your overall experience. Discuss your fasting intentions with your acupuncturist prior to including acupuncture in your program.

Years ago I was teaching a fasting class at the graduate level. Midway through the class I offered the students the opportunity to go through the fasting diet or do a special study (fasting must be voluntary). All but two students chose to do the fast and the program proceeded well through the pre-fast diet and into the juices. On the second day of juices I began getting calls at my office from various students that were experiencing difficulties. By midday I had received about six calls and became concerned that something was wrong. I had never had so many people call me during a fast, even with groups many times larger. I cancelled my afternoon patients and drove out to the graduate college.

When I arrived, I met with the students who were experiencing difficulties. They reported feeling bloated, gassy, and just not very good. Then the first one spoke up that they had all attended an acupuncture class in the morning. Their instructor, noting the many bottles of fresh juice, changed her topic and spent the entire class warning about the dangers of juice for people with the condition of damp spleen. This authoritative condemnation undermined the confidence that these students had in the fasting process. The resultant fear, adrenaline, and uncertainty of their actions led to digestive upset. All of the fasters who had not attended this class were doing fine. All of the fasters that took this class were having problems.

After meeting with me, these students all got back on-track and had successful completion of their five- and seven-day juice fasts. It took one of their professors to break their confidence, but you may be just as susceptible to a mother's concern or friends' criticism. Please remember the general rule of not telling people that you are fasting as their unfounded concerns might undermine your own experience.

I have had many acupuncturists send me patients for fasting or do my programs themselves. It is not universal that all acupuncturists oppose juice fasting. Many understand its safety and its benefits. Many also understand that the physiologic changes that accompany a fast are an ideal environment for the benefits of acupuncture.

Epilogue
Beyond the Fast

The American health-care system is at a critical juncture. While scientific and technological advances have led to new and remarkable changes in some of our medical practices, the cost of medicine, the availability and accessibility of care, and the failure of modern medicine in areas of chronic disease and cancer have all contributed to our current problems.

In 1974 I took part in a GAO (U.S. Government Accounting Office) study of the needs and delivery of medicine in Clackamas County, Oregon. The issues of affordability, delivery, and quality were all present and obvious even at this time. While we have studied and worked to provide better overall health care, we have continued to fall further and further behind. There are some basic flaws in the American approach to health care suggesting that unless we change this approach, we will never find a solution.

One of the most important factors to add to our national health care debate is the principle of holistic medicine. More than the contemporary definition of body, mind, and spirit, I mean holistic in relating societal, occupational, and environmental factors into the individual's health concerns. It is clear that we will never be able to afford the cost of treating the many preventable diseases that we now face. If we can make inroads into areas of domestic violence, prenatal health care, drug treatment programs, health screening programs, and occupational hazards we can create a more productive population with a much less expensive system of disease management.

Preventative medicine means much more than immunizations, mammograms, and blood-pressure screening. It means taking an active role in establishing healthy lifestyles and dietary habits. We have an insidious and unhealthy lobbying influence from food and pharmaceutical industries that look after their own profits and power while evading their responsibility to truth and the public safety. This has led to a system in which economics truly takes precedence over science and public need.

While it is incumbent upon us all to do what we can individually, we have to lead as a nation to a more just world environment. We are one planetary community. The health needs and problems of any nation are no longer "at our doorstep" but are in our "one planetary house." Diseases of Africa and Asia are now American diseases as well. The toxic chemicals of agriculture, banned in some nations, return as food to our own chain. The infectious diseases of one community are just an airplane ride away from our own streets. Our long-term health needs are truly part of a planetary concern.

In practical terms, as American citizens, unless fully insured, few of us can afford the costs of urgent care or long-term needs. There has to be some form of insurance that guarantees the access of Americans to effective medical treatments. It is unfair for a person's life earnings to be consumed by one medical emergency. We do need a disease management system in America, what we call "health care" today. We would benefit by investigating the tiered systems of France and Germany to provide a model that both afforded private insurance and integrated systemwide care.

No "disease management" system will ever be affordable until we see a responsible move of science and the medical industry into preventing disease. We have to question the status quo of agriculture, the food industry, the pharmaceutical industry, and our patent laws regarding new drugs. Until we change the things that we know contribute to our chronic health problems, we will never afford the costs of their treatments.

If we found a method to direct science and research toward ethical needs; to implement government policy based on effectiveness of the policy and not lobbying economics; to significantly reduce the 100,000 American job-related annual deaths; to reduce the socially influenced contributors to disease, illness, and injury, then, as a healthy, working, and active society, health care would be affordable!

Appendix A

Enemas, Problems, and Options

Most people have no problem doing the enemas as outlined in this text. Occasionally, some people have discomfort or are unable to hold the entire two quarts of water. This is most commonly an experience of the first and occasionally the second enemas (before the high-fiber pre-diet materials have all been voided). It is all right to take the two quarts in divided delivery, although almost everyone finds the ability to take a full two quarts by the second or third days. Please take note of the temperature recommendations discussed in the enema section of Chapter 6 because cooling or heating the solution may solve problems of discomfort.

Sometimes the thought of doing an enema is too much. There can be emotional issues that make the physical process of an enema too disturbing. In these cases an alternate to the enema would be either to continue with one teaspoon of psyllium husk powder daily or to eat two to three whole fruits as one meal. These are not as effective as an enema in that the muscles of the colon are not as relaxed throughout this process, but it will eliminate the toxic reabsorption of wastes that will occur on a juice fast with no enemas or fiber support. Reabsorption of toxins can contribute to headaches, fatigue, irritability, and depression.

Liver Tonic and Nausea

The olive oil–based liver tonic can occasionally initiate the sensation of nausea or queasiness. The liver and gall bladder are the primary organs influenced by this tonic. If you have had your gall bladder removed or have a history of intolerance to fats in the diet, you should reduce the recipe to two tablespoons of olive oil, not three. Likewise, if you have other signs of a "sluggish" liver (PMS, chronic headaches, nausea, chemical sensitivity, and fatigue), you may experience nausea with this drink. Again reduce follow-up tonics to two tablespoons, not three, of olive oil.

Quantities for the Pre-Fast Diet

There is a great amount of fiber and bulk in the pre-fast diet. While there are fewer calories than in the typical diet, the volume is much greater than most people consume. It is not essential that you consume every bite of food in the pre-fast diet. Do your best, but a reduced amount of food, especially on the third day, is not going to negatively affect the overall program. If you have very few crunchy vegetables in your normal diet, you may wish to plan a longer pre-fast diet with about two-thirds the total daily volume of vegetable and supplemental fiber.

Reactions to the Juice

Very rarely, someone reacts to carrot, beet, or other vegetable juices. Sometimes the juices are too sweet and it's more a matter of taste than anything else. In this case just dilute the juices. Celery will tend to reduce the sugar content of combination drinks with carrot or beet. If you have allergic responses to any of the juices, try to isolate if it is one particular fruit or vegetable that you are reacting to. If so, simply create other combinations that do not include that particular food. If you seem to be reacting to many different juices or foods, consider trying the Master Cleanser discussed in Chapter 5.

First Bowel Movement

Some people start right up with normal bowel activity the first day that foods are reintroduced. Other people may take one, two, or even more than three days to return to normal bowel activity. As long as you are reintroducing foods as outlined in the reintroduction diet, things will normalize. Don't be concerned if you don't have a bowel movement the first day or two.

Appendix B
Naturopathic Medicine

Naturopathic medicine is an American-born field of medicine following the philosophy *vis medacratrix naturae*, or "let the forces of nature be your medicine." Its origin is credited to a number of American physicians, hygienists, and nature curists who united in the late 1800s to form the new field *Naturopathic Medicine*, circa 1896. Dr. Benedict Lust is popularly called the Father of Naturopathic Medicine and was instrumental in its early identity. Other important contributors to its origin included Dr. Kellogg of cereal fame, Dr. Just (*Return to Nature*), and Father Kneipp, hydrotherapy.

There were many different groups of practitioners that shared a common theme of using nature, diet, and water to reverse the diseases of civilized man. To most of these practitioners, the term *civilized man* was synonymous with living in opposition to nature and natural law. They include the hygienists, the eclectic herbalists, the hydrotherapists, and the nature curists. Most of these early practitioners were M.D.s, as the title N.D. had not yet been created.

From the late 1800s through the early 1900s, there were a number of American colleges that granted the N.D. degree. Most of these graduates practiced throughout the United States under the category of *drugless practitioner*. Some states, like my own home state, Oregon, established naturopathic practice acts in the early 1900s that delineated the naturopath from the broader drugless practitioner. As the category of drugless practitioner left the American law books, the naturopath was often left without a practice act. Today only about fifteen U.S. states have full-practice acts for naturopathic medicine. This number has actually increased in recent years with growing public interest in this traditional form of medicine.

In the early 1900s the American medical system became more defined within a few forms of care. The allopathic (M.D.), osteopathic (D.O.), and chiropractic (D.C.) fields of medicine developed unified approaches of study within each respective group and created medical schools to work within the U.S. education system to grant the respective degrees. By the mid-1900s there were no longer any freestanding naturopathic colleges and the only N.D. degrees were offered within existing chiropractic colleges. In 1952 National Chiropractic College in Illinois granted its last N.D. degree, leaving only Western States Chiropractic College as the last U.S. naturopathic program.

In 1956 Western States granted its last N.D. degree, which led to the immediate creation of the National College of Naturopathic Medicine in Portland, Oregon. Chartered in 1956, this college owes its very existence to the early unpaid work and devotion of Dr. John Bastyr; Dr. Joseph Boucher; Dr. Carl Kennedy Sr.; Drs. Blithing, Stone, and Turska; and others who continued to teach the principles of naturopathic medicine until the college and profession once again found their own feet.

Today National (NCNM) is joined by Bastyr University (Seattle) and the Southwest College of Naturopathic Medicine (Phoenix) as U.S. accredited Colleges of Naturopathic Medicine. Toronto University and University of Bridgeport also have programs that offer the N.D. degree. There are naturopathic programs around the world that teach naturopathic medicine, but these programs do not offer the complete medical studies required to practice as an N.D. in the regulated American states.

Naturopathic doctors are required to take similar studies to all physicians in the areas of human science, diagnosis, radiology, clinical sciences, and therapies. N.D.s have prescriptive privileges and must know contemporary pharmacology for both prescriptions and removal of prescriptions. Naturopaths have extensive studies in clinical nutrition, natural medicines, including herbs and supplements, lifestyle and counseling work, homeopathy, Chinese medicine, and physical medicines including spinal manipulation.

For more information:

The National College of Naturopathic Medicine
049 SW Porter Street
Portland, Oregon 97201-9927

The American Association of Naturopathic Physicians
8201 Greensboro Drive, #300
McLean, VA 22102

Endnotes

Preface

1. Contraris, citing U.S. CDC statistics for cancer mortality, 1972–1996, 6th Annual Cancer Symposium on AHCC (Sapporo, Japan, November 1999).

Chapter 1

1. Herbert Shelton, *The Science and Fine Art of Fasting: The Hygienic System*, vol. III, rev. ed. (Tampa, Florida: Natural Hygiene Press, 1978), pp. 53, 57.
2. Ibid., p. 53.
3. Ibid., p. 49.
4. Ibid., p. 56.
5. "Hygienist, n, an expert in hygiene, or the science of health." Definition from *Webster's New Universal Unabridged Dictionary*, 2nd ed. (New York: Simon and Schuster, 1979). The hygienist movement out of America and Europe advocated raw foods, a vegetarian approach to diet,

and food combining to optimize the hygiene, or internal environment, of the intestinal tract.

6. *Webster's II, New Riverside Dictionary* (Boston: Houghton Mifflin Co., 1984).

7. Sheldon Cohen, et al., "Psychological Stress and Susceptibility to the Common Cold," *New England Journal of Medicine* 325 [9] (August 29, 1991), pp. 606–12.

8. R. Ballentine, *Diet and Nutrition: A Holistic Approach* (Honesdale, Pennsylvania: Himalayan International Institute, 1978), p. 381.

Chapter 2

1. Walt Whitman, "Song of Myself." In *Leaves of Grass* (New York: Random House, Inc., 1891–92), p. 49.

2. Arthur Guyton and John Hall, *Textbook of Medical Physiology*, 9th ed. (Philadelphia: W. B. Saunders Company, 1996), p. 823.

3. Asbestos, as a microscopic structure, possesses very sharp surfaces, which lyse, or destroy, red blood cells, leaving the iron of our RBCs forming a rustlike enclosure of the asbestos. This phenomenon is called hemosiderosis and is very similar to the irritation from sand that leads to the creation of a pearl.

4. Guyton and Hall, p. 843.

5. *Blakiston's New Gould Medical Dictionary*, Harold Jones, et al., eds. (New York: McGraw-Hill Book Company, Inc., 1949).

6. *The Dispensatory of the United States of America*, 25th ed., Arthur Oslo, ed. (Philadelphia: J. B. Lippincott Company, 1955), p. 981.

7. Ibid., p. 1553.

8. United States Environmental Protection Agency, Office of Pesticide Programs, Health Effects Division, "Hazard and Dose Response Assessment and Characterization: Atrazine," 2000 preliminary draft (Washington, D.C.: May 22, 2000).

Chapter 4

1. Paul Ray and Sherry Anderson, *The Culture Creatives* (New York: Harmony Books, 2000), p. 167.

Chapter 5

1. Arnold Ehret, *Rational Fasting*, English translation (New York: Benedict Lust Publications, 1971), pp. 99–100.

2. Kroker, et al., *Clinical Ecology* 2 [3] (Summer 1984): 137–143.

3. Trevor Salloum, N.D., "Therapeutic Fasting." In *The Encyclopedia of Natural Medicine*, Joseph Pissorno and Michael Murray, eds. (Rochlin, California: Prima Publications, 1998).

Chapter 7

1. Fredrick Hollick, *The Diseases of Women: Their Causes and Cure* (New York: TW Strong Publishing, 1858), p. 241.

2. *Webster's New Universal Unabridged Dictionary*, 2nd ed. (New York: Simon and Schuster, 1979), p. 609.

Bibliography

Ballentine, R. *Diet and Nutrition: A Holistic Approach*. Honesdale, Pennsylvania: Himalayan International Institute, 1978.

Cohen, Sheldon, et al. "Psychological Stress and Susceptibility to the Common Cold." *New England Journal of Medicine* 325 (August 29, 1991).

Douglas, Loudon. *The Bacillus of Long Life*. New York: G. P. Putnam's Sons Publishing, 1911.

Ehret, Arnold. *Rational Fasting*. English translation. New York: Benedict Lust Publications, 1971.

Erasmas, Udo. *Fats That Heal*. Burnaby, British Columbia, Canada: Alive Books, 1993.

Gandhi, M. *Diet and Diet Reform*. Ahmedabad, India: The Navajivan Trust, 1949.

Guyton, Arthur, and John Hall. *Textbook of Medical Physiology*. 9th ed. Philadelphia: W. B. Saunders Company, 1996.

Hahnemann, Samuel. *The Organon of Medicine*. 6th ed. Philadelphia: Boericke & Tafel, 1935.

Hollick, Fredrick. *The Diseases of Women: Their Causes and Cure*. New York: TW Strong Publishing, 1858.

Jones, Harold, et al., eds. *Blakiston's New Gould Medical Dictionary.* New York: McGraw- Hill Book Company, Inc., 1949.

Just, Adolf. *Return to Nature.* New York: Benedict Lust Publishing, 1903.

Kellogg, J. H. *Colon Hygiene.* Battle Creek, Michigan: Good Health Publishing, 1916.

Kroker, et al. *Clinical Ecology* 2 [3] (Summer 1984).

Moor, Fred. *Manual of Hydrotherapy and Massage.* Mountain View, California: Pacific Press Publications, 1964.

Nelson, Dennis. *The Tao of Natural Breathing.* San Francisco: Mountain Wind Publications, 1997.

Osol, Arthur, ed. *The Dispensatory of the United States of America.* 25th ed. Philadelphia: J. B. Lippincott Company, 1955.

Pissorno, Joseph, and Michael Murray, eds. *The Encyclopedia of Natural Medicine.* Rochlin, California: Prima Publications, 1998.

Khalsa, Gurucharan Singh, ed. *Sadhana Guidelines.* Los Angeles: Arcline Publications, 1974.

Shelton, Herbert. *The Science and Fine Art of Fasting: The Hygienic System.* Vol. III, rev. ed. Tampa, Florida: Natural Hygiene Press, 1978.

Thich Nhat Hanh. *A Guide to Walking Meditation.* New Haven, Connecticut: Eastern Press Inc., 1985.

Webster's II, New Riverside Dictionary. Boston: Houghton Mifflin Co., 1984.

Webster's New Universal Unabridged Dictionary. 2nd ed. New York: Simon and Schuster, 1979.

Whitman, Walt. *The Leaves of Grass.* New York: Random House, Inc., 1891–92.

Williams, Roger. *Nutrition Against Disease.* New York: Pitman Publishing Corp., 1971.

United States Environmental Protection Agency, Office of Pesticide Programs, Health Effects Division. "Hazard and Dose Response Assessment and Characterization: Atrazine." Preliminary draft. Washington, D.C., May 22, 2000.

Index